Aging Well
Using Eugeria to Stay Young and Healthy

Jean-Paul Lintilhac, M.D.

and

Simone Lintilhac

A Sophie avee ma profonde
sympathie.
J'espère que vous trouverez dans
cet ouvrage, quelques recettes utiles
pour préserver votre energie et
votre bonne humeur.
Très amicalement

Carillon Press
Los Angeles

Photographs on pages 209–212, 223, and 225 are from the private collection of Dr. and Mrs. Jean-Paul Lintilhac

Carillon Press is an imprint of Belle Publishing

Library of Congress Cataloging-in-Publication Data
Lintilhac, Jean-Paul
    Aging well : using eugeria to stay young and
healthy / Jean-Paul Lintilhac, Simone Lintilhac.
—1st ed.
    p.   cm.
    Includes bibliographical references and index.
    LCCN: 99-73043
    ISBN: 0-964-9635-5-8

Interior design and production by Robert S. Tinnon
Cover design by Sparrow Advertising and Design
Editorial assistance by Marcia Aubineau

Belle Publishing
Los Angeles, California
800/627-0750
E-mail: bellepub@earthlink.net

Printed and bound in the United States of America
International Standard Book Number: 0-964-9635-5-8

10 9 8 7 6 5 4 3 2 1

Contents

PREFACE   ix

INTRODUCTION   1

Part I
Preliminary Notions

CHAPTER ONE
What Is Aging?   9
*The Genetic Clock • Catastrophic Errors in the Genetic Code •
Free-Radical Theory of Aging • Hormonal Theory of Aging •
Death Genes? Life Genes? • Low Body Temperature • Denutrition
Without Malnutrition*

CHAPTER TWO
What Is Longevity?   15
*Average Longevity • Projected Life Expectancy versus Life Expectancy
in Good Health • Dysgeria • Retarding and Delaying Your
Physical and Mental Deterioration • Who Is Most Likely to Live Well
Over Sixty?*

CHAPTER THREE
First Survive: A Primary Condition to Eugeria   23
*Causes of Death in Industrialized Countries • Test Yourself Regularly •
Schedule Yearly Tests*

Part II
Risk Factors

CHAPTER FOUR
Toxic Substances   35
*Tobacco • Alcohol • Narcotics • Prescription Drugs • Atmospheric
Pollution*

CHAPTER FIVE
Risk Factors Associated with Nutrition   47
*Excess Weight and Obesity • Malnutrition • The Food Components •
Water • Carbohydrates • Cellulose • Proteins • Fats and Cholesterol*

CHAPTER SIX
Minerals, Trace Elements, and Vitamins   73
*Minerals • Trace Elements • Vitamins • Fat-Soluble Vitamins •
Water-Soluble Vitamins*

CHAPTER SEVEN
Risk Factors Not Directly Related to Nutrition   119
High Blood Pressure • Heredity • Immunity • Stress and Idleness

Part III
Attaining Eugeria

CHAPTER EIGHT
Nutrition   135
*Basic Diet Guidelines • Food Do's • Food Don'ts • Chew! Enjoy! •
Alcolholic Drinks • Recommended Multivitamin, Multimineral
Supplements • Antioxidants • Essential Amino-Acid and Essential
Fatty-Acid Supplements • Prevention (and Treatment) of
Mental Aging*

CHAPTER NINE
General Hygiene and Sex in Old Age 167
Exercise • Activate Your Brain! • Sex and Old Age • Pysiotherapy and Spas

CHAPTER TEN
Treatments for Eugeria 179
Hormone Replacement Therapy for Menopause • Aspirin • Testosterone for Andropause • Growth Hormone • Melatonin • Other Treatments • Short Guide to Supplements for Eugeria • A Typical Day in Eugeria for a Retired Person

Part IV
Looking Young

CHAPTER ELEVEN
The Skin and Its Annexes 203
The Importance of Appearance • Skin Aging • Age-Related Skin Lesions

CHAPTER TWELVE
Keeping Your Face Young 207
The Face • SMAS (Superficial Musculo-Aponeurotic System)

CHAPTER THIRTEEN
Keeping Your Body Young 221
Firm Skin on the Body • Skin Treatment for the Night • Skin Treatment for the Day

CONCLUSION
Why I Believe in Eugeria 229
My Case • Simone's Case

APPENDIX
Nutritive Value of Food 235

INDEX 245

Preface

The goal of eugeria is simple. It provides an accessible, practical guide to what you can do today (not tomorrow, next week, or next year) to age in an optimum way. For the record, I am less concerned with living longer but living more fully. There's more than a grain of truth in that old cliché, "Rather to add life to your years, than years to your life!" My approach requires that we apply—or least to understand—proven scientific principles, but there is also an art to aging well. Drawing from the Greek words *eu* (meaning well) and *geria* (meaning old age), I have developed a program I call *eugeria*. In a nutshell, to pursue a healthy eugeria is to "age well."

Interestingly enough, though I have been studying eugeria since the late seventies, I notice that medical doctors have only taken an active interest in enhancing and supporting the quality of our lives during the past few years. At long last, the medical community is beginning to realize how important it is to focus on preventive care and our long-term well-being. It is a ludicrous notion to only treat people when they are struck down by debilitating or even fatal diseases. Eugeria is more than simply maintaining our health in the "golden years." Its purpose is also to elevate living. We stop growing as early as age twenty, and that's when some of our intellectual and physical capacities begin to deteriorate. Before I send you into the doldrums about this, remind yourself how much we gain as we grow older! We compensate for physical decline after we peak, and with training and experience, our lives can continue to blossom. In many ways our lives become better as we stack up the years.

Introduction

When the mayor of her hometown visited Jeanne Calment—the famous French centenarian who recently died at age 122—on her 100th birthday, he put a hand on her knee and promised to visit again on her 101st birthday. Calment looked at him carefully, then winked and quipped: "And why not? You seem in good shape!" Jeanne Calment's irrepressible spirit and my own accumulating years inspired me to investigate the issue of healthy aging. I have been reading American and European studies on the subject since 1979. I have watched the development of exciting new medical breakthroughs, the emergence of popular trends in treatments and health maintenance, and I have noted the basic, common sense wisdom that has endured both fashion and time. However, through the course of my studies, I have been continually surprised by the animosity existing between mainstream doctors and alternative therapists.

Holistic and alternative therapists believe that nutrition is—more or less—the only effective means to impact our health. For this, conventional medics dismiss these practitioners as quacks and dreamers who subscribe to witchcraft and "unproved claims." You will find in this book that I take the middle path. I use what is useful, and I discard what is not. Alternative medicine offers sage advice in the main, but I am outraged by the hype that often surrounds various new, inadequately tested "magical potions," that profess to cure everything from old age to acne. As for conventional medicine, for too long we have been subjecting ourselves to drug therapy without minding the part we play in our own illness or the long-term toxicity of various treatments. Yet, in the face of life threatening diseases or accidents, radical drug therapy or surgery may be necessary to save your life. I'm all for that.

Nowadays we are bombarded by fantastic claims from every direction. We cannot open a newspaper without reading about some new FDA- (Food and Drug Administration) approved drug purporting to cure disease or an over-the-counter "natural" supplement that purports to prevent it. Allopathic medicine is an enormous industry, yet the alternative market is growing apace. There are great sums of money at stake for both sides. Though I was trained as an M.D., specializing in plastic surgery, I do not believe it serves anyone to be rigidly partisan. The future points to both allopathic and alternative medicine working in synergy for the sake of our health. And I believe that this should be the major agenda of anyone associated with the healing professions.

The most sensible, healthiest way is for us to extract what is best from both approaches. That is why I have researched conventional medicine and alternative therapies in my quest for the means for living better and longer. You will not find miracle cures in this book. But you will find treatments that show practicable rates of improved health and survival.

While I was inspired by Jeanne Calment, I began my research largely in response to my own aging. In 1999 I turned eighty, and I am proud to tell you I am in excellent health. Five years ago, I was surprised by a diagnosis of prostate cancer, but modern medicine has helped me get the condition well under control. However, almost twenty years ago, I was well on course to an old age riddled with health problems. I arrived at age sixty with unhappy hereditary antecedents and a history of risk factors. I decided I wanted to live out my years as best I could. There was so much still to do, so much before me! I resolved to stave off illness and incompetence for as long as I could. I offer this book because I believe my research—using myself as a guinea pig—richly paid off.

I learned to enhance the quality of my life by adding some things to it and dispensing with others. During my long career as a plastic surgeon (I only stopped practicing in 1997), I had ample opportunity to study the exterior dimensions of aging every working day of my life. I learned, for instance, how physical aging impacts one's spirit and total well-being. Coupled with my research and my own lifestyle changes, I was finally moved to begin work on this book.

Our "adult" age ends between fifty and sixty. Historically, we prepare ourselves to enter the "golden age" after age fifty, but nowadays, men and women over fifty are as active as those in their forties a few decades ago. The human life cycle is changing. At best, we feel the need to readjust our lifestyles after age sixty, not after fifty. All the same, it is never too early to prepare for eugeria. The sooner you begin healthy life habits, the richer your later years are likely to be.

While my program is simple, I do not think I'm inviting you to an easy pursuit! If you feel good at fifty, you may not want to bother about changing your exercise and dietary habits. You may resent my suggestion that you submit to a more disciplined life. You may be neglectful about taking your vitamins and antioxidants. You may forget to take the medication your doctor prescribed. But I insist: How you live now will affect your health fifteen years down the line. And take it from me, fifteen years is not that far away. What is difficult to stomach is that nothing—not even my program—guarantees that some accident (either physical or disease-related) will not interrupt your program and dash your best efforts. And then what regrets! I knew a man who followed a strict diet and played a number of sports he did not enjoy because he thought they were "good" for him. He never overindulged and never had any fun. His life was steeped in austerity because he thought that was the way to sidestep disease. Then, at sixty, he was diagnosed with incurable cancer. It was such a tragedy! The truth is virtue does not always compensate for shaky genes. That's why I prescribe good sense and moderation, because there is no question that the sensible adjustments I outline in this book bring overall benefit—that is, improved health, energy, mental capacity, and emotional well-being. But it also allows you to enjoy life as well.

Only severe illness or serious physical or intellectual handicap will transform eugeria into *dysgeria* (*dys*, from the Greek, meaning difficult), and an arduous old age. While my approach is unlikely to cause anyone harm, let me warn you that special circumstances, such as those that involve nursing care, are not within the scope of this book.

In any event, it is easier to be reasonable and practical at sixty than it is at twenty. We're more inclined to rid ourselves of our vices with age, or perhaps, as some suggest, our vices leave us. Whichever way you look at it, for a healthy eugeria, our first—and greatest—challenge is to avoid excess tobacco, alcohol, food, work, and even some sports. Thankfully, for most of us, sexual excess usually takes care of itself as we age, so I will not lecture on safe-sex practices or sexually transmitted diseases. The chapter on sex will offer some guidelines, but I presume you are sensible, once you have overcome your health-defying addictions—which I address in this book. The rest of the program is both straightforward and painless. Your health is in your own hands. Only you can make a difference in your attempt to live better and longer. Some of you may be surrounded by colleagues or family who have no interest in supporting your new, healthy lifestyle. Or you may increasingly bump up against social prejudice, since society doesn't always take kindly to senior citizens. Whatever your circumstances, if you commit to a healthy eugeria, you will be strengthened to tackle whatever fortunes and misfortunes your later years bring you.

I have wanted my wife, Simone, who has been my closest collaborator for forty-five years, to participate in this book and give her advice on subjects she is familiar with, subjects on which she may have a slightly different opinion or some more practical information to share with us. She will represent in this book the voice of common sense as opposed to the more theoretical, and sometimes difficult to understand discourse I have a tendency to use due to my scientific background.

So don't be surprised to find Simone's comments in a different and more familiar tone at the end of many chapters. She has been invited to speak freely on the subjects nearest to her heart. I hope this will be a refreshing adjunct to what I have to offer.

And now, since she has been invited, I will let her speak for herself and tell you a little more about her life with me.

SIMONE

The reader may ask what my qualifications are to intervene on the subject at hand. To the dear reader, I may answer: "I'm not sure" . . . perhaps my age (soon to be seventy-five), my permanent concern to maintain my good health and looks, my experiences of living and working beside my husband and keeping in contact with many of our patients for over forty-five years . . . or simply that I enjoy being a part of a good discussion with my husband. So, dear reader, with my husband's blessing, comment I shall!

I have always defined myself as my husband's wife. What would the feminist movement read in that? Personally I don't care, for I am my husband's wife, and it suits me perfectly. My life has changed completely since I married him in 1953 in Casablanca. I was a Parisian traveling in Morocco, and he was a young plastic surgeon just back from the United States where he had studied for two years and was in the process of opening a clinic to practice his art, the first and only one in the country. It was over a year before we finally wed. Since our wedding, I have been a wife and worked professionally with my husband at the clinic, receiving the patients, briefing them on what to expect, and encouraging them before and after treatment.

My husband was very active in the hospital, where he practiced mostly reconstructive surgery, and in his private clinic, where patients would flock to undergo his successful cosmetic surgery.

After thirteen wonderful years in Morocco, pushed by some more ambitious projects, we decided to move to Paris in 1965 and open a luxurious private clinic in the center of town. There my husband practiced only cosmetic surgery, having abandoned any hospital appointment.

The success of his surgery in Paris attracted many European and American patients. Ten years later, in 1975, working fourteen hours and operating ten hours a day until late into the night, and paying excessive taxes, my husband, who had some problems with his health, decided to take no chances and to slow down.

He asked me if I would like to move to Tahiti. We both loved Tahiti, where we had spent several vacations since 1963. I agreed. I must add that in Tahiti a French diploma is valid, and last but not least, Tahiti is a haven where there is no income tax. (Taxes had become excessive in France.) So we moved to Tahiti by Christmas 1975 and opened a new clinic. Due to my husband's reputation (he was cited among the eight most famous plastic surgeons in the world), patients poured into Tahiti from all over. Television shows from the United States and Australia included the clinic as one of the main reasons to visit Tahiti.

When he arrived in Tahiti, at fifty-seven and in questionable health, my husband became increasingly interested in the study of aging and the many ways to fight it. At our clinic, we introduced the most up-to-date antiaging treatments available at the time, such as cell therapy promoted by Dr. Paul Niehans from Switzerland, injections of Gerovital introduced by Dr. Anna Aslan in Romania, and also the amenities and physical therapies that are available in the most modern spas, including thalasso therapy and proper diet. Experimenting on food supplements and antioxidants, my husband came to the conclusion that they were more active and less expensive ways than these injections to fight the aging process. He abandoned completely the cell therapy treatment that necessitated a complicated organization to bring the living cells to Tahiti. Finally, continuing his research on new discoveries and important ways to fight the aging process, he pursued and tested different treatments on two of his closest and most favorite participants as test subjects . . . himself . . . and me!

Part I

Preliminary Notions

CHAPTER ONE

What Is Aging?

H umans consist of cells, water, and fibers. And cells, water, and fibers make up living tissue. While the function and fabric of living tissue is a miracle in itself, one remarkable property is that in the nucleus of our cells, a coded message—our genetic blueprint—delivers instructions to proteins to build up our bodies. In other words, our genes are the medium that configures the proteins that keep us alive. There are three basic routes into the theory of aging, and each has their validity.

THE GENETIC CLOCK

The most common theory of aging is centered on the way the passage of time modifies the genetic program. Like passengers on a train, we are subject to a journey for which the tracks are already in place. The journey begins at conception, takes us through the changes of birth, childhood, adulthood, and old age toward our destination, which is ultimately death. We are passive "victims" of our own built-in genetic time line, because our cells can only divide and reproduce a finite number of times. The basis of this theory rests on the systematic shortening of strings of nucleic acid attached to the ends of the chromosomes that live in the nucleus of every one of our cells. These strings are called *telomeres*, and each time our cells divide, they are diminished. Once the telomeres are completely reduced, the cells become damaged and begin to die off.

CATASTROPHIC ERRORS IN THE GENETIC CODE

A second theory proposes that aging is the result of "catastrophic errors" by which, on our journey through life, our genetic code is altered and cannot be corrected. There is always some idiosyncrasy involved in the reproduction and repair of our genetic code anyway, but subscribers to this theory believe that the sudden flaws that cause cell damage are the things that cause death.

FREE-RADICAL THEORY OF AGING

The third theory concerns the activity of free radicals in the body. Let me give you some background: Atoms, comprised of protons and electrons, make up the molecules that make up our cells. A collection of active electrons spins around the nucleus of the atom, which is composed of protons. The active electrons are coupled in pairs, but due to various circumstances, on many occasions, they split from each other. This leaves single, bachelor electrons known as *free radicals*, which embark on a frantic quest to pair up again. Their reactivity causes damage to cells and allows for disease and deterioration of the whole body. Particular free radicals give the medical community cause for concern. They are known as *oxygen-based free radicals*, consisting of two atoms of oxygen and a bachelor electron. In this form, they indiscriminately attack any molecule in our bodies—either they abandon one of their electrons or they seize another from a neighboring molecule. The result is a chain of events in which new free radicals are generated that behave just as reactively. In the end—and in a few nanoseconds—our cell membranes and genetic codes are significantly damaged. The chain reaction can end in different ways: At best, the free radical joins another free radical, and the molecule is stabilized with two paired electrons. Otherwise, enzymes produced by our bodies or free radical scavengers—antioxidants—are occasionally able to provide the free radical with a single electron without harm to themselves. Antioxidants are most often vitamins that, after neutralizing the free radicals, become slightly reactive themselves. Later, they lose their reactivity and are actually regenerated to their original form by the presence and action of other vitamins. Though this is a minor introduction to antioxidants and vitamins, rest assured your understanding will broaden through the course of this book. I discuss them at length. Free radicals are also produced during normal oxidation that occurs as we breathe. This is not all to our detriment, because the oxidation of certain nutrients creates the energy that keeps us alive. Also, our own white blood cells actually produce free radicals to battle bacteria and the viruses that try to invade our bodies. These useful free radicals are deactivated by the enzymes superoxide dismutase, catalase, and glutathione peroxidase—all of which are produced inside us. What's most important for us to know is that health-defying free radicals are produced accidentally by radiation or toxic agents, such as tobacco and alcohol, industrial pollution, and high cholesterol. These are things we can do something about. First, we can adjust our lifestyles to suppress the cause, and we can embark on a program of antioxidant supplements. I discuss this more later, but first, let me introduce you to a few other—rather radical—theories on the process of aging and extending life.

HORMONAL THEORY OF AGING

The hormonal theory of aging was put forward some fifty years ago by a scientist named Denkla. He pointed to the existence of an internal hormonal biological clock that included DECO (degressive consumption of oxygen hormone), a "death hormone" that originates in the pituitary gland, the regulator of all our hormone production. According to Denkla, the death hormone retards the efficacy of the receptors to our other hormones, and so prevents them from functioning at all. For example, the hormone thyroxin is important to our metabolism, but if DECO develops unchecked, our bodies are prevented from absorbing and using thyroxin. What's more, DECO creates more free radicals. These damage our genetic code and accelerate aging. While Denkla's theory is no longer popular, there is no question that hormones play a significant role in health and in aging. Nowadays, doctors prescribe hormone replacements such as growth hormones, sex hormones, DHEA, and melatonin to combat and retard the symptoms of decline. There is no doubt that hormones, and the hormone receptors, need our attention. For example, when the hormone insulin is not absorbed by the hormone receptors, we suffer the effects of insulin resistance, such as high and harmful blood-sugar levels (hyperglycemia and hyperinsulinemia), raised blood-fat levels, high cholesterol levels, atherosclerosis, and diabetes. Though I talk about hormones throughout the course of this book, I do not believe we can build a theory of aging on hormones alone. Quite simply, what we inherit by way of genetics and the impact of free radicals are just as significant.

DEATH GENES? LIFE GENES?

All over the world, modern researchers are trying to isolate the genes that cause aging in an attempt to discover those that prolong life. The futuristic desire is to extract the "death" genes and enhance the "life" genes, so that we can set ourselves up for unprecedented longevity, and even eternity. The theory is as follows: If cancer cells are immortal, why can't creative, immortal, "life" cells exist as well? As I write this, however, not only are these radical studies extremely new, but as yet, they're unproven. Therefore, until we have conclusive research and a satisfactory methodology to create immortality, I suggest we turn our attention to supporting our bodies and using the tools we understand and already have now.

LOW BODY TEMPERATURE

Some say that if we lowered our body temperatures, then we would live longer and in good health. This theory rests on our knowledge that flies, certain fish, and iguanas live longer when their body temperatures are sustained at cool levels. But the temperatures of these creatures—known as *poikilotherms*—are determined by their environment. We humans are different. We are *homeotherms*; our systems are set up to sustain body temperature, and we are only slightly affected by the cold and heat that surrounds us. In fact, it is almost impossible to lower our temperature for any length of time. So to my mind, though this approach is still debated, it is not practical.

DENUTRITION WITHOUT MALNUTRITION

The well-known Dr. Roy Walford, of the University of California, is one of those rare theorists who practices what he preaches. He fasts two days a week, limits his caloric intake through the rest of the week, and takes enough supplements to ensure what he calls "undernutrition without malnutrition." In 1986, Dr. Walford reduced the caloric intake of rats and mice and discovered that the animals not only lived longer, but were less prone to cancer. So he applied his discoveries to his own life. I cannot deny that his findings are interesting, but I am not entirely enamored of Walford's program. For many of us, the effort of following such a strict regimen might be disheartening to the point that most of us would give up. What is more, I'm not convinced that embarking on a reduced calorie program after age fifty does not adversely impact our physical health. I prefer a more practical program. Eugeria is about enhancing the quality of our lives. Why add on years if they are filled with stressful and excessive restrictions?

SIMONE

This section, I feel, is theoretical and difficult to understand for someone who does not have basic knowledge of biology, of genes, and of DNA. This is the case of most older people who were educated at the time when these structures were not yet discovered; this is also my case. Nevertheless, I am thankful to you for trying to explain this in simple words. As you like to say, "Could we let them die completely ignorant?" This is also true for free radicals, but I agree we must have some knowledge of these unpaired electrons and the damage they can do to the cell membranes and our DNA, to understand how antioxidants work for the protection of these vital structures. The experimental ways to extend longevity do not seem very practical, although Roy Walford's method of reducing caloric intake might be worth trying for someone who has faith in science to the degree of abnegation necessary to embark on this experience that will deprive him or her of some of the joys of life.

CHAPTER TWO

What Is Longevity?

W hen Jeanne Calment—the impish French woman I mentioned in the introduction to this book—died, she was over 122 years old. She was, officially, the oldest human being alive. Every animal has its own maximum life expectancy, for example, tortoises can live up to 200 years. Humans are unlikely to exceed 120 years. Calment's longevity was not only awesome, it was highly unusual.

AVERAGE LONGEVITY

In trying to project how long we may live, we must account for our "average longevity," a statistic that is determined by our race and sex, not to mention our historical context. Back when the United States was founded, life expectancy at birth was only about thirty-five years. It reached forty-seven years in 1900, jumped to sixty-eight years in 1950, and steadily rose to seventy-six years in 1991. In 1991, life expectancy was higher for women (seventy-nine years) than for men (seventy-two years). The reason for the increase is due to the progress of hygiene and medical therapies, especially vaccinations and antibiotics. In industrialized nations, progress affected the rate of infant mortality, which is no longer a major concern in our modern world. It wasn't long afterward we discovered that twentieth-century medical breakthroughs influenced a progressive lengthening of the average longevity, especially during the last fifty years. When I first began research-ing aging, I noticed that every common census calculated length of life, but never considered a quantifiable quality of life. That is when I came up with the idea of eugeria. The term was inspired by the illness *progeria*, a condition in which young children age at an alarming rate and often die before they reach twenty. Con-versely, eugeria is about dying young, but as late as possible!

PROJECTED LIFE EXPECTANCY VERSUS LIFE EXPECTANCY IN GOOD HEALTH

Finally, in the mid 1980s, a grouping of around one dozen teams interested in demographic studies—known collectively as REVES, the "Reseau Esperance de Vie en Santé (Network of Life Ex-pectancy in Health)—introduced a new index of measuring life expectancy in good health. Since then, the French have calculated life expectancy in two different ways: First, they measure aver-age life expectancy, and second, they try to measure life expectancy in good health. In other words, they realized that as we age, qual-ity of life is as important a factor as clocking up years. Between 1981 and 1991, total life expectancy without incapacities increased from 60.8 years to 63.8 years for men, and from 65.9 years to 68.5 years for women. Now, I am inclined to calculate that the period of eugeria begins at age sixty. Therefore, with these statistics in mind, I figured that in 1991, the average French man could ex-pect to sustain his good health for 3.8 years after his sixtieth birth-day, and the average French woman could sustain her good health for a short 8.6 years! How depressing! Having come to your well-earned retirement, all you have is three to eight years to enjoy it. Wouldn't it be sensible to try and extend the vitality of a sound body? By committing to a healthy eugeria, we can significantly re-duce the gap between our projected life expectancy and our life expectancy in good health. I project that we could add at least

9 healthy years for men, and 12.5 years for women. In other words, while our goal begins with enhancing our years, a healthful eugeria increases our chances of adding years to our lives, too.

DYSGERIA

Let's turn our attention to the alternative to eugeria. Sudden death not withstanding (brought on by acute disease or accident), the prospects facing senior citizens can often be gloomy. If not eugeria, life after sixty can be marked as a period of dysgeria. (Remember? From the Greek *dys* for difficult, *geria* for aging.) Physical and mental handicaps such as arthritis, depression, Alzheimer's, Parkinson's, and heart disease, as well as the final phases of cancer, are just a few of the predicaments plaguing an unhealthy old age. Finally, loss of good health means loss of independence, and many men and women end up in institutions or relying heavily on their families long before they must. I do not undervalue the care and support offered by residential hospitals and homes, but I encourage you to retain your independence for as long as possible.

RETARDING AND DELAYING
YOUR PHYSICAL AND MENTAL DETERIORATION

Prolong and lengthen the vigorous years. Live your life in eugeria. To live life in eugeria is to pursue a profitable activity or to fully enjoy a freely chosen and organized retirement. The only effort involves reducing your risk factors, preventing the onset of disease by engaging in early warning procedures, and embarking on a simple program of a few life-enhancing supplements and drugs. The savings you realize by preventing disease and embracing good health will undoubtedly offer a greater return than the adjustments, expenses, and efforts you invest. Researchers know that certain life choices and life circumstances affect life expectancy. We might begin our program by understanding the stressors and comforts we have—and have had—in our lives. They have come up with some interesting statistics.

WHO IS MOST LIKELY
TO LIVE WELL OVER SIXTY?

Researchers have determined that the inactive, the unemployed, and the retired die earlier than those who are active and working. The probability of inactive people dying between fifty-five and sixty-five is 40 percent higher than the probability of active people dying in the same age range. That figure hovers at a mere 17 percent. Cultural circumstances affect our life expectancy: A laborer at thirty-five years of age has the same risk of dying as a skilled worker at forty-five and professionals and executives at age fifty-three. Marriage, or at least some form of family life, seems to protect men, as the probability of a man dying between thirty-five and sixty is determined as follows:

Married: 15%
Single: 20%
Divorced: 31%
Widowed: 35%

Professionals and executives increase their longevity if they live in an urban environment. For those living and working in a big city, the mortality rate is reduced; on the contrary, for unskilled laborers living in rural areas, their projected life expectancy is enhanced. A cramped and too-small apartment can take years off your life, and so can renting your living quarters: Statistics show that homeowners are inclined to live longer than tenants. For women, issues of cultural circumstance, education, social environment, and professional activity do not affect longevity in the

A LONGEVITY QUIZ

The following quiz is designed for individuals to project their own life expectancy.

Beginning with the base number of 72, add or subtract according to the guidelines that follow:

Personal Data	*Base number*	**72**
Men	Subtract 3	_____
Women	Add 4	_____
If you live in an urban area with more than 500,000 inhabitants	Subtract 2	_____
If you live in a town with less than 10,000 inhabitants	Add 2	_____
If one of your grandparents lived until 85 years	Add 2	_____
If all four of your grandparents lived until 80 years	Add 6	_____
If one of your parents died of stroke or heart attack before age 50	Subtract 4	_____
If a parent or sibling has or had cancer, heart disease, or childhood diabetes before age 50	Subtract 3	_____
If your cholesterol level exceeds 4 g without treatment, or 3 g with treatment	Subtract 4	_____
If you have a university degree	Add 1	_____
If you have a post-graduate degree	Add 2	_____
If you are 63 years or older and still working	Add 3	_____
If you are a man living with his spouse	Add 5	_____
If you are a woman still with her spouse	Add 2	_____
If you live alone, for each decade you are over 25 years		
Men	Subtract 5	_____
Women	Subtract 1	_____
If you are left-handed	Subtract 3	_____

A LONGEVITY QUIZ, *continued*

Lifestyle

If you work behind a desk	Subtract 3	_____
If you work necessitates physical effort	Add 3	_____
If you exercise vigorously (tennis, jogging, swimming) at least 5 times per week for at least one-half hour	Add 4	_____
If you exercise two to three times a week	Add 2	_____
If you sleep more than ten hours a night	Subtract 4	_____
If you are naturally tense and aggressive	Subtract 3	_____
If you are easygoing and relaxed	Add 3	_____
If you consider yourself happy	Add 1	_____
If you are unhappy	Subtract 2	_____
If you have been fined for speeding in the past year	Subtract 1	_____
If you smoke 2 packs of cigarettes per day	Subtract 8	_____
If you smoke 1 to 2 packs per day	Subtract 6	_____
If you smoke 10 to 20 cigarettes per day	Subtract 3	_____
If you drink 1 to 2 whiskeys or half a liter of wine per day	Add 3	_____
If you drink only occasionally	Add 1	_____
If you are a heavy drinker	Subtract 8	_____
If you are overweight by 44 pounds or more	Subtract 8	_____
If you are overweight by 33 to 44 pounds	Subtract 4	_____
If you are overweight by 11 to 33 pounds	Subtract 2	_____
If you are a man and have annual health checkups	Add 2	_____

A LONGEVITY QUIZ, *continued*

Lifestyle, *continued*

If you are a woman and have an annual gynecological checkup	Add 2	_____
If your diet consists of mainly simple foods, fruits, and vegetables, as opposed to meat and fatty foods	Add 2	_____
If you supplement your diet with vitamins and antioxidants	Add 4	_____

Adjustments for Age

If you are between 30 and 40 years old	Add 2	_____
If you are between 40 and 50 years old	Add 3	_____
If you are between 50 and 70 years old	Add 4	_____
If you are over 70 years old	Add 5	_____

My life expectancy: (Copy last entry)   ——

SOURCE: Originally compiled by Robert F. Allen and Shirley Linde and published in their book *Lifegain* (Human Resources Institute Inc., 1981). I have added a few of my own modifications.

way they do men. Nontraditional family life is less serious for women as bachelorhood is for men, and widows have similar life expectancy levels as married women.

From this quiz I'm glad to see that the risk factors and the favorable factors are the same in France and in the United States. And why not? After all, we are civilized human beings subjected to the same hereditary, psychological, and biological inferences. There are a number of controllable factors. You may not easily choose between being a farm laborer or a lawyer in a big city. But you can watch what you eat and the number of toxins you choose to ingest. Eugeria, while it primarily improves the quality of life, certainly lengthens your life as well.

SIMONE

Dear J. P.:

Being happily married to me for forty-five years will add at least six years to your life expectancy in the longevity quiz.

CHAPTER THREE

First Survive:
A Primary Condition to Eugeria

Eugeria is neither an alternative nor an antidote to conventional medicine. I offer no substitutes for scientific practices, particularly where major ailments such as heart disease or cancer are implicated. Here is a program to support your good health and counter the manageable effects of decline. At the same time, while I offer no radical cures for any major diseases, I guarantee that this program will help to prevent them.

CAUSES OF DEATH IN INDUSTRIALIZED COUNTRIES

There are a few common causes of death in industrialized countries. Here are the statistics for adults:

Cardiovascular disease	32.5%
Cancer	18.6%
Stroke (vascular cerebral accident)	13.0%
Fatal accident	5.0%
Infectious disease	3.3%

Heart disease, cancer, and stroke continue to be the top three causes of death in the United States. Leading causes of death differ by age. In 1995, accidents were the leading cause of death for people between one to four, five to fourteen, and fifteen to twenty-four years of age. HIV infection was the leading cause of death for those aged twenty-five to forty-four years. Cancer was the leading cause of death for those aged forty-five to sixty-five years of age and over.

The causes of death and ranking for 1995 are listed as follows:

Diseases of the heart	737,563
Malignant neoplasms	538,455
Cerebrovascular diseases	157,991
Chronic obstructive pulmonary diseases	102,899
Accidents and adverse effects	93,320
Pneumonia and influenza	82,923
Diabetes mellitus	59,254
HIV infection	43,115
Suicide	31,284
Chronic liver disease and cirrhosis	25,222

Cardiovascular Disease and Stroke

Note that cardiovascular disease and stroke are a factor in more than half of all deaths! There is some good news, however. Both cardiovascular disease and stroke are brought about by the same risk factors. Not only are these risk factors self-induced, but also they are managed and treated most easily. These are the health conditions in which we, as individuals, play the greatest part. They are the conditions we can do the most about.

What's more, vascular problems usually announce themselves by way of early warning, and you are likely to experience uncomfortable symptoms, such as chest pain or numbness and pain down your left arm, which will alert you and your doctor to a potential condition. Unfortunately, cancer is insidious and—particularly in it's early stages—can only be detected by regular medical examinations, some of which necessitate sophisticated laboratory testing, such as MRI, mammogram, angiogram, CAT scans, and assorted blood tests.

Cancer

Americans over sixty-five display ten times the risk of developing cancer than anyone younger. In fact, a whopping 60 percent of cancers occur in persons after that age. While this is unsettling, cancers that are detected early are most successfully treated, whatever your age. Statistics show that 40 percent of patients who benefit from early detection are likely to survive for at least five more years. Older people often neglect systematic testing for cancer, not realizing the risk they are taking. The last thing you must do is ignore your chance for developing this ugly disease. Besides embarking on a program of wellness, I also prescribe a healthy relationship with your doctor, who will likely advise regular mammograms and colonoscopies. These tests are imperative for a vibrant eugeria.

TEST YOURSELF REGULARLY

For systematic medical management after age sixty, even if you do not experience any particular and alarming symptoms, I recommend the following:

1. *Once a month you should, by yourself, test your pulse and blood pressure.* Do not begin this procedure after rigorous exercise. With your left-hand hanging down, follow the line of the thumb and place your right index and middle fingers above the base of the thumb on the underside of your left wrist. If you apply soft pressure to this area, you will detect the "beat" of your pulse. Using a stopwatch or a clock with a second hand, count the number of "beats" in a minute. At rest, a normal count adds up to around sixty beats per minute. If your count exceeds seventy-five (at rest) or measures below fifty, this is cause for concern and time to talk to your doctor. Likewise, you should consult your doctor if you notice any irregularities in the rhythm of the pulse.

As with the pulse, we normally test our blood pressure at rest.

I like to use a small finger device called a blood-pressure monitor that is sold in most pharmacies for around $100. Before you begin using the device systematically, I suggest that you standardize your readings with those of your doctor. This is because results are often affected by the way you hold the machine in relation to your body. Once you have done that, and you are doing the test alone at home, begin the procedure by first sitting down. Once you are settled, place your index finger in the cylindrical chamber, put your hand in your lap and follow the simple directions displayed on the machine. You will receive two readings: The first measures your systolic pressure (corresponding to the contraction of your heart muscle), and the second reading measures your diastolic pressure (corresponding to the relaxation of your heart muscle). Average systolic measurement range between 130 and 140 and upward of 150 is cause for concern. Similarly, average diastolic measurements range between 70 and 90. Over 90 must be checked out. If your readings diverge too far from the norm, the best thing to do is talk to your doctor.

2. *Weigh yourself.* You may have a good inkling of your ideal weight, but confirm your thoughts with a medical professional. Further, once you have established that ideal, be sure to monitor unusual increases or decreases in weight. In eugeria, it's best not to fluctuate. Even if you were a few pounds heavier or lighter than you would like to be, you would do better to sustain your weight than embark on any foolhardy diets. I will offer dietary recommendations later on in this book.

3. *Women should conduct manual examinations of their breasts.* With the right hand held flat, firmly explore the breast clockwise and counter-clockwise in a circular motion, mindfully searching for any unusual lumps. In addition, sweep the hand in an upward motion from the bottom of the breast to the top, and from left to right. Once the left breast has been fully explored with the left hand held flat, repeat the procedure in regard to the right breast. If any unusual lumps in either breast is detected, the doctor should be contacted.

4. Examine your skin for any new growths, changing moles (otherwise known as nevus) or discoloration.

5. Learn to tune into your body, and monitor the way you feel physically. While you will sense minor physical and emotional fluctuations from one day to the next, call your doctor if you experience any abnormal change or unusual discomfort.

SCHEDULE YEARLY TESTS

Once a year, you should:

1. *Schedule blood tests.* Including a complete blood count, chemistry, enzymes, and PSA (a test for prostate cancer for men.) Laboratory reports provide an all-important early-warning system for a variety of diseases. Remember, the earlier any ailment is treated, the greater your opportunity for optimum recovery.

2. *If needed, schedule a urine examination.* While your doctor will often search your blood tests for indications traditionally detected in urine samples, urine samples are a less invasive—though less sophisticated—means to testing for some conditions.

3. *Schedule an examination with a cardiologist.* He or she will measure your blood pressure and—by means of a stethoscope—monitor the health of your heart and blood vessels. Your cardiologist will also conduct an EKG (electrocardiogram), during and after controlled aerobic effort (to raise your heart rate), with a view to analyzing the strength and efficacy of the energetic currents emitted by your heart. Alternatively, your doctor might ask you to submit to an echocardiogram, an ultrasound device that projects an image of the heart on a monitor. This way, he or she can detect for any irregularities in the heart muscle, as well as its valves and cavities. In addition, you may be required to undergo an echographic Doppler exam, to test the health of your veins and arteries.

4. *Visit your dentist.* At least once a year schedule an appointment with your dentist to check the potency of your mastication, the health of your gums, and whether your teeth are still well-

rooted. Among other conditions your dentist will check for are poor mastication and paradentose—loose teeth and inflamed gums. These are dental issues typically associated with advancing age. The better the health of your gums and teeth, the better you are able to digest your food.

5. *Every woman must schedule an annual mammogram with her gynecologist.* In 1994, 1,721,700 women had been diagnosed with breast cancer, which accounts for 39 percent of all cancer diagnosed in women. Early detection is the first hope of survival. Most doctors recommend women begin yearly mammograms as early as forty. If you have no problems with X ray, and you have a history of breast or any other cancer in your family, I definitely advise annual mammograms. When breast cancer is found early, the chances of survival are as high as 95 percent! No doubt yearly testing is the least you can do.

6. *Even post-menopausal women should continue to monitor their gynecological health.* Besides regular breast examinations, I strongly advise you never let up on your yearly pap smears. Further, if you follow a program of hormonal replacement therapy, then you should visit your gynecologist at least every six months.

7. *Prostate exams.* Similarly, while the PSA test is the most efficient method for detecting prostate cancer, as an extra precaution, men can be examined by an urologist for enlarged prostate or benign tumors.

8. *Intestinal exams.* At least every two years you should schedule an examination with a gastroenterologist. By using ultrasound devices, he or she will conduct abdominal echographies and explore your colon and stomach with colonoscopies and gastroscopies. These tests are used to detect incipient stomach and colon cancers, ulcers, polyps, and various other intestinal diseases.

9. *Heart and lung exams.* If, at your annual checkup, your cardiologist did not conduct a radioscopy—that is, an X ray providing images of your heart and lungs—now is the time to schedule a test. Lung cancer is the most common cancer afflicting men, and

for women the incidence of this killer is increasing apace. Both your cardiologist and your general practitioner are able to prescribe thoracic X rays to search for lung cancers, chronic bronchitis, and a number of other respiratory disorders. If your doctor detects any irregularities, then he or she can refer you to a lung specialist.

10. *Eye exams.* Every two years you should consult an eye specialist, not only to check your vision and adjust your glasses but also look for incipient cataract, glaucoma, or macular degeneration.

A Word for Conventional Treatments

If any disease is detected through any of these channels, allow your doctor to treat you with conventional medicine and the appropriate drugs. While eugeria promotes the proper use of vitamin supplements, healthy diet, and lifestyle, these are preventive measures, not life-saving treatments. Eugeria is designed to help you stave off life-threatening illness, but it does not claim to treat coronary problems or cancer. In other words, my program does not replace conventional medical care; rather, it proposes the sensible use of your doctor's attention. It goes without saying that if you experience irregular or disquieting symptoms between regular checkups, then contact your doctor as soon as you can. Remember: First survive! Then launch into and enjoy your eugeria.

Risks to Survival

Before illness comes risk factors, and your doctor is more than likely to advise you to eliminate them. These are various habits and behaviors that undermine prolonged good health, which are determined by your medical history and heredity.

Bottom-Line Risk Factors for Cardiovascular Disease
Any or all of the following may lead to cardiovascular disease:

- Any amount of tobacco consumption.
- Excessive consumption of alcohol: My research shows that 40 to 50 g of pure alcohol per day is the upper limit. That translates into no more than four glasses of wine per day or no more than two whiskeys.
- Obesity and inadequate nutrition: If you are more than ten pounds overweight, then you are already at risk. However, even if your weight is normal, and you consume too much fat, then your risk is comparable to, if not greater than, those with minor obesity. Refer to the chapter on fats and cholesterol in the Nutrition Section for my guidelines on fat consumption.
- Diabetes: Often associated with excess weight and tobacco.
- High cholesterol: Associated with diet.
- Hypertension: High blood pressure, associated with stress and heredity.
- Sedentary lifestyle and stress: Due to lack of exercise or, conversely, inadequate rest.

Bottom-Line Risk Factors for Cancer
The following contribute to cancer: Tobacco, alcohol, carcinogenic by-products of industrial activity, such as asbestos, air pollution, and tar; as well as radiation from the sun, nuclear waste and X rays. Your intake of excessive fats and nitrates from fertilizers, the latter of which find their way into the food supply, may also be a factor. For this reason, it is best to select organic fruit and vegetables whenever you can. Again, your personal risk factors are determined by your medical history and heredity.

Accidents
Believe it or not, the greatest risk to older people on the road is not themselves, but accidents caused by the reckless behavior of

young adults—most often young men. However, an older person's risk is increased by his or her own performance. As we age, our performance and reactions inevitably deteriorate or at least slow down. Of course, alcohol is an exacerbating factor, as is the effect of some medications. Be sure you discuss the issue of driving with your doctor whenever you are prescribed any new medication, over-the-counter or otherwise.

SIMONE

Here, for once, I completely agree with you. I have read books on aging, staying young, reaching 100 years, but as much as they recommend diet, exercise, vitamins, antioxidants, hormones, even meditation, no one mentions the absolute necessity of recognizing cardiovascular problems or incipient cancer and treating them with conventional medical treatments. I noticed that most people reaching the respectable age of ninety are survivors who have suffered a life-threatening infectious disease, an accident, a heart attack, or a light stroke. I'd like to give you the example of our old friend, a great businessman, who suffered a heart attack at seventy-six and underwent five bypasses on his coronary arteries. Although he was very serious about walking three to five miles every day and following the prescribed diet and medication, he had to submit again to heart surgery at eighty-three and finally died of heart insufficiency at ninety. In the meantime, he was active, going to the office every day in a state of pretty well-preserved eugeria.

Another example of surviving in eugeria is the case of former French President François Mitterand, who already had prostate cancer when he was first elected in May 1981 (this was revealed only several years later). He was reelected for a second mandate of seven years in May 1988, still with his prostate cancer, for which he underwent surgery and multiple treatments. Nevertheless, he performed his duties as an active president. He died one year after the end of his second mandate at age eighty. I agree with you that surviving is the primary condition of eugeria, and that we should submit to regular checkups as you recommend.

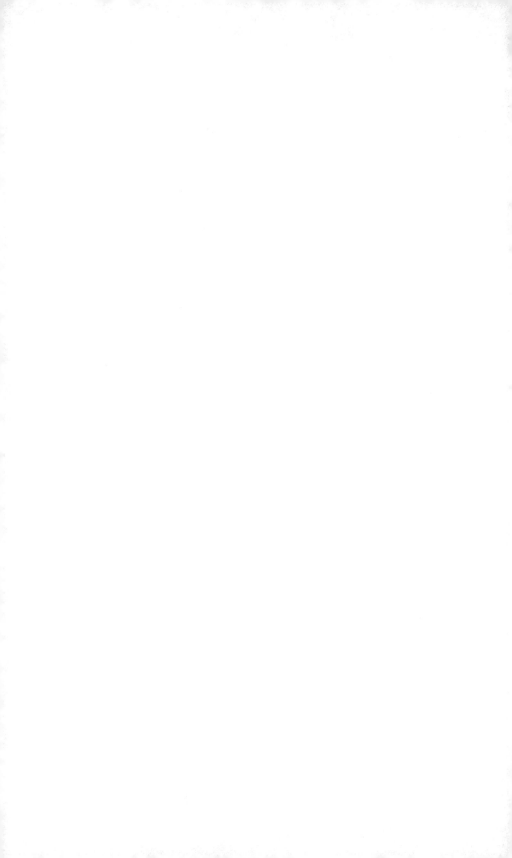

Part II

Risk Factors

CHAPTER FOUR

Toxic Substances

Without question, the distinct risk factors of alcohol, tobacco, and various other toxic substances contribute to the deterioration of organs, cells, and molecules—the physical demise often attributed to aging alone. The first imperative of eugeria is to eliminate or reduce such toxic behaviors, often self-inflicted, to a level where they cease to be harmful. Interestingly enough, there is a point where some of these so-called "risk factors" can become beneficial. For instance, mild consumption of alcohol can support a healthy heart and contribute to the prevention of diabetes. I'll discuss this in due course. A second—and equally manageable—tier of risk factors is associated with nutrition. Obesity, or a compromised metabolism leading to certain disorders, can be caused by the different food components just as deficient consumption of vitamins and minerals can lead to disease. Finally, we must face the risk factors of hypertension, heredity, immune-system deficiencies, lack of exercise, and stress. The following chapters take a look at them all. You can begin by eliminating—or at least controlling—your exposure to toxic substances. A number of toxic substances contribute to disease and death.

TOBACCO

Statistics gathered in the United States show that, in spite of antitobacco campaigns, one out of every six American deaths is due to tobacco-related disease.

Similarly, in France, tobacco is responsible for 30 percent. of deaths by cancer: Of these cancers, 87 percent is of the lung, 85 percent of the larynx, 65 percent of the mouth, and 40 percent of the bladder. Tobacco also contributes to 21 percent of deaths by heart attack, 18 percent by stroke, and 82 percent of death by obstructions of the bronchial tubes.

Tobacco contributes to a litany of ills. Not only does it advance certain cancers, but it is also known to aggravate others. It also contributes to sterility, hyperthyroidism, and complications associated with protruding eyes. It is responsible for doubling the risk of noninsulin-dependent diabetes between ages forty and seventy-five, as well as significant decreases in muscular strength and bone mineral density, which in turn leads to postmenopausal osteoporosis. It goes without saying that tobacco damages our lungs and respiratory functions.

As a cosmetic surgeon, I am acutely aware that the blood supply to smoker's skin is significantly decreased in contrast to that of nonsmokers. Without adequate blood supply, the skin actually dies—we call it *necrosis*. When I perform a face-lift on a smoker, I know that the "flaps" created by extensive "undermining" of the skin are unlikely to receive sufficient blood. Therefore, I watch out for the dead, blackened skin that sloughs off from the face, leaving unsightly defects. The wound can heal itself, but most often I must schedule the patient for skin-grafting surgery. Smokers look older. Smoking accentuates facial wrinkles because free radicals in smoke attack the skin. Further, the act of smoking—that is, the habitual contraction of the muscles around the lips caused by sucking on cigarettes—causes wrinkles all by itself.

If you smoke and also lay, work, or play sports in the sun, know that smoking exacerbates the ill effects of sun radiation, just as the sun increases the ill effects of tobacco. There is more! In American research into 151 domestic fires, of the fires causing death of people in a household, 31 percent of the fires were caused by smokers. I think it is safe to assume the statistics for death by fire caused by cigarettes is greater for smokers over age sixty. Quite simply, older smokers are more inclined to fall asleep with a cigarette or forget about a butt burning in an ashtray.

If the myriad studies explaining the ill effects of smoking on your health and good looks are insufficient to prompt you to quit, let me encourage you by saying that several studies show it is never too late to make the effort. Your health will improve whenever you stop. In fact, it is as important for older adults to quit as it is for youngsters. For those over sixty, I would say it is imperative. Remember that there is a notable lengthening of life expectancy in industrialized nations. Why throw away your opportunity to enjoy an enhanced quality of life—nothing less than the achievable goals of eugeria? It is never too late: If you are over sixty, and continue to smoke, there is still plenty of opportunity to avoid and reduce bronchiopulmonary diseases and improve and regenerate your fitness and strength.

If you do not smoke but live, work, or associate with smokers, it is in your best interest to persuade them to quit. The dangers associated with "passive smoking" are almost as severe as active smoking itself. If you cannot get them to quit, at least ask them to smoke outside the premises or far away from you. Having begun my case against smoking, dare I suggest it, but there are a few minor benefits to be garnered from cigarettes. Believe it or not, one is a decreased risk of Alzheimer's disease. A few particular studies show that in families where Alzheimer's is a factor in heredity, family members who smoke seem to contract the disease a tad later than those who don't.

Additionally, smoking may be favorable in cases of ulcerative colitis, a disease of the colon marked by ulcers and bleeding. However, I must warn you that the benefits in these instances point to the nicotine found in tobacco, not the tar, which remains highly toxic and dangerous. For those wanting to explore nicotine as an antidote to these diseases, nicotine patches are a viable alternative to cigarettes. Truthfully, there is no good reason for you to smoke.

If you have never smoked or have stopped smoking, bravo! Otherwise, I pray that you quit as soon as you can.

Why Should You Quit? How Should You Quit?

There is no way around it, whatever method you choose, you will need some willpower, and to engage that, you first need motivation. If fully appreciating the effects of smoking on health is not enough motivation, then I am not sure what is. If you have ever watched a friend or family member die from lung cancer, emphysema, or any other smoking-related disease, you will understand what I mean.

If you are prone to any of the risk factors associated with heart attack, high cholesterol, or high blood pressure, your continued use of cigarettes will greatly increase your chance of attack. Any doctor will tell you: Quit smoking, and you are on your way to saving your life.

If the prospect of good health, or even avoiding a tragedy does not persuade you, consider a few of the following: Smoking is slavery and unworthy of any civilized being. Smoker's breath is grossly unpleasant. Morning cough is both uncomfortable and tiresome. Cigarette burns in your clothes and household linen are unattractive and annoying. Believe me, you will appreciate these seemingly frivolous arguments the minute you quit!

If you struggle to control your addiction yourself, then there is no reason not to seek professional help. Millions do! Nowadays, there are thousands of successful programs available to assist smokers in becoming healthy ex-smokers.

The Nicotine Patch and Nicotine Gum
This skin patch is applied in digressive doses for an average period of three months and significantly eases the brutal withdrawal

symptoms, which often cause smokers to give in and light up. Similarly, you can chew nicotine gum when your withdrawal symptoms feel intolerable. While these two products serve the body's craving for nicotine, they help break the habit of smoking and work very well in the early stages of quitting. As a new quitter, you can regulate your use of the gum according to your own needs.

Acupuncture
When it is applied in a particular way, the ancient art of Chinese acupuncture has a sedative effect on the body that reduces the psychological factors that drive smokers to cigarettes. That is, by reducing your levels of anxiety, depression, and chronic anger, acupuncture can enhance your willpower to quit.

One last word: Quitting is not easy, and it is important to enlist the cooperation of your loved ones to support you in this process. How many spouses and loved ones, exasperated by the tantrums and temper of the recent ex-smoker, have held up a pack and cried, "For goodness sake, smoke! I can't take your mood swings anymore!" While tempers might flare for a couple of months, in the end, emotional harmony is more likely to prevail. With the end of foul breath, smoky clothes, and holes in the bed sheets, relationships might even improve in the long run, rather than deteriorate!

ALCOHOL

Compared to tobacco, alcohol is more difficult to pin down as a risk factor. While no one can reasonably recommend any use of tobacco, we now know that a minimal daily consumption of alcohol is actually beneficial to health and eugeria.

The highly respected Framingham study—which began in 1948 and continues today—was established to study and monitor the health of a particular community. Consistently, researchers in the study reported that a moderate use of alcohol—they mention 30 to 50 g per day—is healthier for the heart than excessive consumption or total abstinence.

Similarly, the Framingham study also revealed that alcohol protects against noninsulin-dependent diabetes—in effect, moderate drinkers have a 40 percent greater chance of avoiding noninsulin-dependent diabetes than teetotalers.

That is why, doctors today generally recommend 30 to 50 g of alcohol daily for adult men, and 20 to 35 g for women. If you are over seventy, I suggest you follow the guidelines for women, because the body's ability to metabolize alcohol decreases with age. Further, certain alcoholic beverages are more healthful than others. See Part III, Chapter 8, for further discussion.

Alcoholism

Let me distinguish between festive, convivial drinking and the addictive disorder of alcoholism. There is a pathological limit, which should not be exceeded. If you crave alcohol and experience physical and mental malaise, if your need is not satisfied, then you are dependent, and most likely in trouble.

The Causes of Alcoholism

First of all, you should know that biologically, some people are at greater risk for alcoholism—or any addiction—than others. Heredity and social environment also play their part. Nowadays, we are pretty certain that a propensity toward alcoholism runs in families, but social, cultural, and individual psychological influences can be equally compelling. Modern psychologists point to fixation engendered by disruptions at a child's oral stage of development. In France, a baby's bottle is called a *biberon*, and drinking alcohol is often described as "biberoner."

Alcohol fills spiritual emptiness, numbs loneliness, masks low self-esteem, and feeds the fantasies we may have of ourselves. Sadly, these good feelings only last for as long as intoxication allows, and the downside of "coming down" and impaired motor functions are the depressing sideeffects of excessive consumption.

The worst case scenario is death. Acute alcoholic intoxication traverses between simple euphoria and dangerous delirium.

With four or five grams of alcohol in the blood, you are in danger of falling into a coma and dying, either by accident, or by toxification. Still, let me distinguish between alcoholism and visible intoxication. If you drink every day but are never drunk, that does not mean you are not an alcoholic. Quite a few alcoholics never seem drunk, but they are just as addicted and just as much at risk. Conversely, if you had too much champagne at your granddaughter's christening and embarrassed your wife, that does *not* mean you have a problem—only the problem with your wife! Still, excessive consumption is dangerously toxic and causes lesions within your body.

Health Hazards Associated with Alcoholism
Your pancreas, which helps in digestion and the control of blood-sugar levels, becomes damaged and inflamed. Alcoholics often develop acute pancreatitis, a painful disease that can cause death.

Your liver, essential to your metabolism, often develops cirrhosis, a degenerative disorder in which healthy cells are destroyed and replaced by fibrous tissue. While death from untreated cirrhosis can be inevitable, deterioration is slow and can take years. What is more, cirrhosis negatively affects other organs and bodily functions, and so the afflicted often suffer long periods of extreme discomfort as they slowly deteriorate. The reason why alcoholics become violent, indifferent, jealous, and inconsistent is because alcohol affects the central nervous system, the source of which is located in the brain. At worst, untreated subjects deteriorate into dementia. In addition, the peripheral nervous system is

affected by inflamed nerves, atrophied muscles, and lost sensitivity most likely caused by liquor's destruction of the body's B vitamins. That is not all: Alcohol alters our fat metabolism (especially
high triglycerides) which may promote coronary heart disease,
and many studies suggest that osteoporosis is induced by or exacerbated by excessive alcohol, too.

Alcoholism in People over Sixty

As you safely enter eugeria, you will be relieved to know that alcoholism is most prevalent in people between the ages of forty and fifty,
and it decreases after age fifty. One reason for this is, quite simply,
few alcoholics survive after fifty. They either wind up with severe
psychiatric disorders or die at the hand of alcohol-related diseases.
The other, more comforting, reason is that spontaneous cessation
occurs in many cases. Studies show that the mean consumption of
alcohol in the general population reaches its maximum before age
fifty and decreases later. However, if you are an alcoholic, do not
take this as a sign that you will quit without effort somewhere down
the line, and you can drink yourself to oblivion while the going is
good. In the majority of cases, addiction is addiction, and the disorder does not desist until the addict commits to treatment.

Occasionally, older people increase their consumption and give
in to alcoholism in later years. Perhaps they were moderate drinkers
throughout their lives, but with pain, health problems, loss, and bereavement occurring later in life, they turn to liquor as a panacea.
Alcoholism is more than a bad habit, it is an illness. Fortunately, it
can be treated at any age. In fact, it is more successfully treated in
older people. Programs such as Alcoholics Anonymous (AA) propagate complete abstinence, insisting that it's illusory to ever hope
for moderate use in the future. One single glass can spiral into a
dangerous relapse. A few modern programs are less stringent. While
these may be useful, AA, historically, has had enormous success, and
the new programs have not yet been tested by time.

While quitting is one aspect of healing, supportive care by one's doctor and family are essential components to sustained sobriety. If you have a history of alcoholism, or if alcoholism was a factor in your family, it is probably wise to abstain from all liquor. For those not at risk, moderate consumption is not only safe, but advisable! However, for those over sixty, I suggest you decrease your consumption as you continue to age.

NARCOTICS

You may have read that limited marijuana use is helpful for relieving pain associated with cancer. To my mind—especially if you have an advanced cancer—there is no reason not to obtain relief with one or two joints. Similarly, if your doctor prescribes it, go ahead and take morphine. Why suffer unduly? Having said that, there is no recreational drug in existence that benefits health. If, at age sixty plus, you still indulge in narcotic delusions—or as I call them, tragedies—put down this book and go ahead. Get on with it. There is no point in pursuing eugeria until you have quit.

PRESCRIPTION DRUGS

Yes, prescription drugs have their place among risk factors, especially as far as older people are concerned. When you are older, your eliminatory functions, particularly your liver and kidneys, slow down significantly. Therefore, prolonged use of prescribed medications can accumulate in your system and become toxic, even deadly. Carefully read the side effects associated with any drugs you are taking and know that they might be increased and exacerbated in your advanced age. Not only should you remain vigilant to your progress under certain prescriptions, but insist that your doctor keep an eye on things too. If you notice any of the following symptoms, inform your doctor, who should adjust and regulate your medicinal dose.

Problems Associated with Over-Prescribed Medications

Barbiturates (such as sleeping pills), antidepressants, and beta-blockers—prescribed for hypertension and arrhythmia—can cause confusion, disorientation, impaired memory, and dyskinesia, an impairment of motor function. Tranquilizers and drugs prescribed for angina can also cause dizziness, which often leads to accidents, either inside the home or on the road. All drugs potentially cause gastrointestinal problems, especially the anti-inflammatory varieties prescribed for arthritis. Diuretics, prescribed for hypertension and water retention, and beta-blockers can contribute to urinary disorders, incontinence, and abnormal retention of waste.

ATMOSPHERIC POLLUTION

The major air-polluting health hazard is ozone (a molecule made of three atoms of oxygen, O_3), a component of photooxidant pollution, which is mainly produced by exhaust fumes and natural compounds transformed by ultraviolet radiation from the sun. Ozone is more abundant in summer and normally peaks in the afternoon. Many major cities recognize ozone as a health hazard and inform their citizens—via news broadcasts—when air pollutants reach dangerous levels. Older people are particularly vulnerable to bad air, especially those with chronic respiratory disorders, such as asthma.

If you are at risk, stay home, close your windows, and rely on air conditioning during peak ozone and other toxic conditions. Also, avoid intense exercise, and never neglect your prescribed treatment program. When conditions worsen, you might increase your dosage.

If you work around or drive diesel-driven machines, you should know that diesel engines produce a gaseous waste known as *acido particular pollution*. This can cause severe inflammation of the lungs.

Finally, free radicals are produced by pollution, and they alone cause pulmonary lesions. During pollution peaks, there is a known increase in mortality, especially among the vulnerable. Still, while air pollution is an obvious hazard to a vibrant eugeria, it is more important you attend to your overall health and medical care. Exposure to ionizing radiation and various chemicals (benzene, asbestos, vinyl chloride, arsenic) increases the risk of cancer.

SIMONE

Remember when you stopped smoking for health reasons? I stopped at the same time to support you. I could not do less.

Thank God, we are not alcoholics, but we like alcohol and never forget our daily ration of red wine.

We never took, nor even tried, any narcotics.

When we moved to Tahiti, we also moved to cleaner air.

CHAPTER FIVE

Risk Factors Associated with Nutrition

The more I learn about health and medicine, the more I realize how that old adage "we are what we eat" makes excellent sense. Our food affects us, both physically and emotionally. It bolsters our health, on the one hand, and plays a role in disease on the other. Without question, food is an essential component of a healthy eugeria. This chapter introduces you to nutrients, calories, and the categories, composition, and proportions of various foods—the very building blocks to understanding nutrition and making healthy food choices.

Food can be a risk factor. For example, excessive consumption can lead to obesity that is, in itself, a major health hazard. Also, many people suffer from food allergies, for example to sugar or dairy products. If a conventional doctor cannot identify the cause of your "malaise," you may do well to consult a nutritionist. Most foods can be classified as proteins, carbohydrates, or fats. Depending on one's individual metabolism, each can cause problems: For example, excess fat contributes to obesity and high cholesterol; excess protein contributes to uremia, a kidney malfunction; and too many carbohydrates can cause diabetes. Watching your intake is important, but so is monitoring the effects of certain foods on your system.

EXCESS WEIGHT AND OBESITY

Obese old people are rare, because most have died of complications associated with their obesity before reaching eugeria. Maintaining a healthy body weight depends on the balance between your caloric intake versus caloric expenditure: In other words, you should eat only as much as the energy you expend in physical labor, exercise, or even fighting disease. Since we tend to expend less energy as we age, our daily intake of calories should be reduced accordingly. For older people, this reduction is natural, but still it is important to keep an eye on your weight.

Who Is Overweight?

The National Institute of Health uses a measurement called body mass index (BMI) to determine whether someone is overweight. To calculate body mass index, multiply weight in pounds by 703. Then divide that result by height in inches, squared. A person, male or female, who is 5'1" and weighs 132 pounds would have a BMI of 25 and would be considered overweight. At 158 pounds, the person would have a BMI of 30 and be considered obese.

As of June 1998, the rules changed and the federal guidelines that were 27.3 BMI for women and 27.8 BMI for men to be considered overweight became 25 BMI for both sexes, adding some 37 million people to the 60 million already overweight Americans (55 percent of the population).

It was also recommended to measure the waist circumference (due to fat around the inner organs): thirty inches in men and thirty-five inches in women signify an increased health risk in those with a 25 to 34.9 BMI.

Look at the following scale, which illustrates how excess weight affects mortality rates:

- For a weight in excess of 15 to 25 percent, mortality increases by 16 percent.
- For an excess of 25 to 35 percent, mortality increases by 30 percent.
- For an excess of 35 to 50 percent, mortality increases by 54 percent.

- For an excess of 50 to 74 percent, mortality increases 130 to 182 percent.

Complications Associated with Obesity

High blood pressure and high cholesterol are just two of the major complications associated with obesity.

Surprisingly, high cholesterol is not always a given in overweight people. Also, it can be a problem for thin people, as cholesterol is essentially a symptom of fat intake and genes. Do not assume your cholesterol levels are safe if you are slim. High blood pressure and cholesterol increase the risk of atherosclerosis, a serious disease characterized by lesions and narrowing of your arteries by cholesterol deposits. At worst, atherosclerosis can lead to heart attack, or even stroke.

Risk of Heart Attack

Overweight adds pressure and strain on the heart muscle, which requires it to work harder. Quite simply, if your heart is forced to work too hard, you risk a heart attack.

Diabetes

Late diabetes is four times more frequent in obese people than those of normal weight.

Difficult Surgery

It is more difficult to operate on obese people because of the inhibiting layer of fat, and therefore, as a result of surgery, obese people die twice as often as those of normal weight.

Rheumatism

Obese people are more likely to suffer from rheumatism. This is because of their compromised metabolism and the pressure of their weight on their spine, hips, and legs.

General Discomfort

If you are, have ever been, or know anyone who is obese, you will appreciate that breathlessness, profuse sweating, and sensitivity to heat are also common—and chronic—discomforts associated with unchecked obesity.

Losing Weight

There is no question that many health problems and discomforts are avoided or prevented by a progressive and controlled loss of weight. However, in eugeria, you should also know that weight fluctuations are detrimental to health, as well as damaging to the skin, bones, and heart. If you have difficulty losing the last five or ten pounds to reach your ideal weight, go easy on yourself. Rather than desperately swinging between losing and gaining them, why not learn to live with those few extra pounds. In France, we have a saying, which roughly translates as, "Over forty, you have to choose between your buttocks and face!" So what if a few pounds leave you self-conscious about the size of your rear end. Losing them might mean you lose the looks in your face. There is always a trade off! In eugeria, we must accept certain things, such as accepting that older bodies are different from young ones (see Table 5.1). Or we can resort to cosmetic surgery, which I discuss later.

After age sixty-five—more or less—there is a decrease in muscular and an increase in fat mass, so we generally gain weight, up to eight to twelve pounds, until we reach age seventy. After that, our weight is inclined to stabilize. In a perfect world, you would reduce your caloric consumption and drop up to ten pounds during this fifteen-year period, until you reach the ideal weight you may have been at age twenty-five. Note I suggest your "ideal" weight. If you were overweight or underweight in your twenties, obviously you should take that into account!

Table 5.1 Caloric Intake for Older People

Women over 75
    Sedentary: 1,600–1,800 calories per day
    Active: 1,800–2,000 calories per day

Men over 75
    Sedentary: 1,800–2,000 calories per day
    Active: 2,000–2,500 calories per day

MALNUTRITION

Sometimes, older people living in poverty, living alone, or living in institutions suffer from malnutrition. This common risk factor is not often addressed, yet it is simply (though not easily) treated by a well-balanced diet. The first cure for malnutrition includes sufficient amounts of essential vitamins, minerals, and trace elements. Also, an important antidote is to introduce supplements to a meager diet. Besides balanced meals, vitamins, minerals, antioxidants and the like, the inclusion of amino and fatty acids is essential to restore low blood-protein levels and to rebuild a weak body.

THE FOOD COMPONENTS

Proteins, carbohydrates, and fats have their own metabolic anomalies which, if recognized and understood, are best managed by diet. Quite simply, nutrition is about consuming a variety of foods, of which certain components are essential to the smooth functioning of our bodies. Other components, though they are not nutrients, are also necessary parts of our diet. Most nutrients are not assimilated directly and are subjected to digestion until the essential elements are absorbed by our bodies. We need water, energetic matter (proteins, carbohydrates, and fats), vitamins, essential amino and fatty acids, minerals, and trace elements to live. And we need cellulose (fiber), as a mechanical aid to digestion.

WATER

We are composed of 70 percent water. In fact, life originated in water and cannot exist without it. Although the sensation of thirst usually tells us we need water, occasionally, and especially in older people, the impulse to drink is sometimes impaired. It is imperative that you drink enough water, especially when you are taking various drugs. The extra liquid makes you urinate more, to dispel any unnecessary toxins from your sensitive system. Diuretics and cortisone put older people at risk for dehydration, as does hot weather and sweating. Be sure to drink plenty of water every day, especially in summer. Severe dehydration is considered a medical emergency, and you could die in two days if you are not treated immediately.

Healthy nutrition is the foundation of a healthy eugeria. More than that, it is the foundation of keeping alive. Read on to understand what healthy nutrition means.

CARBOHYDRATES

Carbohydrates make up the bulk of fruits, vegetables, and grains. By definition, they are molecules composed of carbon, oxygen, and hydrogen and are classified as sugars, starches, and glycogen. Sugars and starches are broken down into monosaccharides (such as glucose, common in grapes), disaccharides (such as sucrose, found in sugar cane), and polysaccharides (such as the starch in potatoes or corn).

Glucose and fructose are absorbed directly from our intestine into the blood, but complex sugars and starches must be broken down first. It is important for you to know that these take a while longer to reach the bloodstream.

Once absorbed, our bodies transform 110,000 glucose molecules into one large glycogen molecule, which is subsequently stored in the liver and muscles for future conversion into energy.

Daily Carbohydrate Intake for Eugeria

In people over sixty, the daily carbohydrate intake should be:

If you are sedentary: 250 to 350 g
If you are active: 320 to 480 g

Several hormones metabolize carbohydrates. The most important of these is insulin, which is secreted by the pancreas. Insulin's job is to help glucose penetrate, and thus feed, our cells.

Hypoglycemia-Hyperglycemia

Excessive insulin depletes the level of glucose in the blood, and some people suffer from hypoglycemia (low blood sugar), a common condition caused by this excess. If you have sudden slumps in energy, shakiness, and occasional disorientation, especially if you haven't eaten, you may fit the profile for hypoglycemia. As we get older, our capacity to metabolize glucose decreases, though you should know that hyperglycemia (high blood sugar) varies amongst individuals of the same age.

Diabetes

Diabetes in older people occurs when the efficiency of insulin is reduced to the point where glucose is inhibited from entering our cells. Diabetes in older people is a crucial health risk. Insulin-dependent diabetes is genetic in origin, and is identified as a health issue at an early age. Still, if you manage your insulin-dependent diabetes well throughout your life, you can survive just as well in eugeria.

Noninsulin-Dependent Diabetes

Noninsulin-dependent diabetes is most often identified after age forty-five, and the risk increases by two or three times after age fifty-five. As your age increases, your risk increases, especially if you are prone to carrying excess weight.

If you break out in boils or suffer from infections that take too long to heal, you may find that diabetes is part of your problem. These are the ailments that most often lead doctors to diagnosing diabetes in people over age sixty-five. However, if you habitually submit to regular blood testing, then your condition will be detected before these skin ailments occur. As always, one rule applies. Early diagnosis is best. Diabetes is serious. It can trigger heart problems. In fact, in many cases, it is difficult to discern whether vascular illness is brought on by high cholesterol or the incidence of hyperglycemia.

Preventing and Managing Diabetes

The best prevention for diabetes is to control your food intake. First lose weight. Also, control your carbohydrate consumption, especially simple, quickly absorbed sugars such as candy, cakes, and fruit that create a toxic blood-sugar "rush." Rather, you should opt for complex carbohydrates, such as potatoes and pasta. These are composed of polysaccharides and starches, and their absorption into the body is more controlled and prolonged. If you smoke, your risk of diabetes is greatly increased. Believe it or not, tobacco used by thin people—yes, more than obese people—multiplies the risk of diabetes by three.

Surprisingly—given its sugar content—two to four glasses of wine per day is a favorable weapon against late-onset diabetes. Studies show that those who drink moderately have a 40 percent reduced risk of contracting the disease as compared to teetotalers. If a controlled diet and regular exercise does not cure you, there are always classical treatments available. However, I advise you to vigilantly monitor any treatment approach. Some treatments induce hypoglycemia, which is particularly dangerous for older people.

Complications Associated with Diabetes

You must seek out treatment, because the complications associated with diabetes are deadly. These include stroke, heart attack, blindness, gangrene, kidney lesions, and finally, diabetic coma. Diabetics also run the risk of functional handicaps that greatly hamper the quality of their lives, such as rheumatism, neurological disorders, and cataracts. While these symptoms are less severe, there is absolutely no question that they are unpleasant.

The first defense against diabetes is regular blood testing to monitor the glycemia, or glucose levels, in your blood—you will be asked to deny yourself food for at least six hours before blood is drawn. Normal levels stabilize around 1 g per liter, but in older people, 1.3 g is most often acceptable. Otherwise, any divergence from these levels requires further tests and, possibly, treatment.

CELLULOSE

Cellulose is fiber. And there are two types of fiber that are essential to digestion: Insoluble fiber (like bran) and a more gelatinous soluble fiber. Both varieties are abundant in fruits and vegetables. Foliage-eating herbivores, such as cows and giraffes, are able to digest cellulose with the aid of an enzyme called *cellulase*, but we humans cannot absorb fiber into our bodies. However, we need it; its role in digestion is imperative to our good health.

Once your food has been broken down—by chewing and with the help of the digestive juices in the stomach—fiber serves to transport the "bolus" of food through your intestine and out the other end! Fiber is essential to America's war against constipation!

More than that, fiber separates the various nutrients in this bolus and exposes and presents them to the digestive enzymes that absorb their goodness into your blood.

Colon Cancer and Diverticulitis

Fiber contributes to the prevention of colon diverticulitis. This is a condition in which the diverticula, tiny sacs on the colon wall, become inflamed. At worst, diverticulitis can lead to colon cancer.

Recent studies reveal that certain insoluble fibers are particularly effective in preventing diverticulitis and colon cancer. If you suffer from constipation or obesity, 20 g or more of insoluble fiber per day (say in bran) can help you enormously. Further, if you suffer from high cholesterol, you will find that 8 to 16 g of soluble fiber (apples, celery, and leafy vegetables) are an excellent antidote. Soluble fibers found in abundance in fruit and vegetables stimulate the proliferation of the intestinal wall. Fermented in the colon, these fibers generate a lot of volatile fatty acids that are immediately absorbed by the cells of the colon. However, they do not protect against colon cancer.

PROTEINS

After water, living matter is made up of more protein than any other substance. In fact, the simplest organisms—such as viruses and bacteria—are composed of nothing more than one bulky protein molecule. By definition, proteins are complex chemical structures composed of nitrogen-rich amino acids. Our genes are constructed from proteins. And an individual protein, along with its constituent amino acids and our genetic propensity, is the component that sets one human apart from every other human. Proteins are indispensable to nutrition for a variety of reasons: First, we lose a certain amount of nitrogen every day, and this can only be replaced by our intake of proteins. More importantly, a number of amino acids are indispensable for creating the proteins that compose living matter. These are called *essential amino acids*. They cannot be manufactured by the body, but must be consumed.

Essential Amino Acids

Scientists have identified around twenty different amino acids. About one half of these are essential, and I list them as follows, along with the recommended daily intake of each in Table 5.2.

Principal Sources of Proteins

Some primary sources of protein include: meat; poultry and eggs; fish; crustaceans (such as lobster and shrimp); other shellfish (such as oysters and clams); wheat; wheat germ; barley and other cere-

Table 5.2 Daily Recommended Intake of Amino Acids*

L-tryptophane	0.50 g
L-phenylalanine: (phenylalanine can be substituted	2, 20 g
by thyrosin at least up to)	70 to 75%
L-lysin	1, 60 g
L-threonine	1, 00 g
L-methionine: (methionine can	2, 20 g
be covered by cystine at least up to)	80 to 89%
L-leucine	2, 20 g
L-isoleucine	1, 40 g
L-valine	1, 60 g

*These guidelines apply only if you also receive sufficient nonessential amino acids through your food intake.

als, such as bread; legumes, such as lentils and dry beans; nuts, such as almonds and peanuts; dry yeast.

Each food source contains different amino acids in variable proportions. A protein's composition—or "aminogram"—is integral to its nutritive value. Normally, proteins cannot pass through the intestinal wall but are broken down into amino acids by our digestive enzymes. After they have been broken down, they are absorbed by the intestinal cells and from there are drawn into the bloodstream. Generally speaking, the richer a food is in amino acids, the richer the source of life creating protein it contains for our bodies. Further, when they are not building proteins, amino acids contribute to the pH balance—that is, the composition of acid and alkaline balance—in our blood. Amino acids are a source of energy, which we measure in calories. Generally speaking, one gram of protein converts to four calories. As the proteins combust, they produce a by-product of waste—urea—which is passed through the kidneys and eliminated in urine.

Uremia

If you have any kidney malfunction, then urea can build up in your blood. This leads to uremia, a condition of extreme toxicity, which, if left untreated, can end in coma and death. Nowadays, as an antidote, external artificial kidneys are used to extract high levels of toxins and nitrogen from the blood. Modern procedures can be dangerous, however. And for that reason, I encourage you to plan a long-term preventive approach. You can fight uremia and the degeneration of kidney efficiency without resorting to drug therapy or surgery. In eugeria, I suggest you keep an eye on your diet, and be sure to eat proteins on a daily basis. We need to eat them, and regularly. They are necessary to compensate for lost nitrogen from our bodies and to supply indispensable—and life-creating amino acids. But in case of kidney problems, your intake of proteins should be kept to a minimum (around 30 g).

How Much Protein Per Day?

I recommend a daily intake of around 50 to 80 g of protein per day. It's not so difficult.

One-half gallon of milk will set you up for the day;
150 g turkey provides half your allowance;
150 g chicken = 32 g protein
150 g beef = 44 g protein
150 g fish = 35 g protein
150 g peanuts = 40 g protein (but also 850 calories)

It is always best to choose proteins low in fat because you should decrease your fat intake. Therefore, I suggest you think twice before choosing red meats, and learn to enjoy more fish, cereals, fat-free milk products, and legumes.

Uric Acid

Warning: If you enjoy offal, such as sweetmeats, brains, liver, and kidneys, be aware these foods contain nucleoproteins, containing nucleic acid, which transforms into uric acid. Excess uric acid in the blood deposits in tissues around joints and can result in gout and kidney stones. A yearly blood test should alert your doctor to uric acid levels in your blood. 70 mg of uric acid becomes cause for concern, and your doctor will advise you what to do next.

FATS AND CHOLESTEROL

You have probably heard of "artery goo" and "artery sludge." Though unattractive, these popular terms aptly describe atherosclerosis or clogged arteries—the unhappy result of an abnormal fat content in your blood. If left untreated, atherosclerosis invariably leads to heart attack and stroke. Fats (technically described as lipids) are composed of carbon, hydrogen, and oxygen, and you should know two things about them. One, they are insoluble in water. And two, because fats are rich in hydrogen and relatively poor in oxygen, they are highly combustible. This means that one gram of fat translates into nine calories—more than double the caloric value of carbohydrates or protein.

Cell membranes are mostly composed of fats and are almost impenetrable. This way, the cell membranes have a dual purpose: First, they control the absorption of minerals and nutrients brought to our cells via the blood. And second, they protect our cells from the water that makes up the compartments between the cells. Excess water would flood the cells, and literally, drown them.

The alimentary fats are divided into three groups:

1. The simple fats made of the association of fatty acid and glycerol; they are the triglycerides.
2. The esters of sterols composed of molecules of fatty acids and a derivative of cholesterol.
3. Complex lipids like lecithin that participate in the formation of lipoproteins.

Only fatty acids and glycerol are absorbed directly. Digestion transforms the more complex lipids into fatty acids and glycerol.

A number of fatty acids are not produced by our bodies but must be ingested. They are the essential fatty acids, also known as polyunsaturated fatty acids.

Polyunsaturated, or Essential Fatty Acids

Polyunsaturated fatty acids dissolve, transport, and eliminate excessive cholesterol from the body. They also act as a vitamin (vitamin F), which aids the health of the skin. There are two families of essential fatty acids.

Omega-3 oils

The omega-3 oils are found in all green plants, especially algae. They only solidify below −73° Celsius, and for this reason, they accumulate in fish that inhabit cold seas. With a different composition of fat, these fish would freeze! The omega-3 oils are especially important for the healthy development of our brains and eyes.

Omega-6 Oils

The omega-6 oils solidify at −20° Celsius and are found in corn, soy, and sunflower oils, as well as animals fed with corn and grains. While omega-6 fatty acids play a part in the development and function of our brains, their intake should be restricted. Why? Omega-6 oils are prone to creating free radicals, those reactive, bachelor electrons that damage the cells and allow for disease.

Saturated, or Nonessential Fatty Acids

Saturated fatty acids solidify at body temperature. Therefore, you can assume they are found in land animals, hence in meat and milk products. Saturated fatty acids (along with monounsaturated fatty acids, see below) are also known as nonessential fatty acids.

Composition of Natural Fats

Just to complicate things, no natural fat is composed of one fatty acid or another. In fact, most are composed of a mixture of all. Further, mono- and polyunsaturated fats are composed of variable proportions of omega-3 and omega-6 oils. Still, we categorize oils as saturated or unsaturated depending on the dominant percentage of whichever fat is found within them.

Monounsaturated Fatty Acids

Polyunsaturated fatty acids are defined by the presence of several double links in their composition. Monounsaturated fats are defined by a single double link. Saturated fats have no double links. All you really need to know is that monounsaturated fats are better for cooking, and you should choose this variety as much as you can. This is because under heat, monounsaturated fats are not destroyed to the same extent as are polyunsaturated fats. Polyunsaturated fats are converted to artery clogging saturated fats when you cook them. See Table 5.3.

How Much Fat Should You Consume?

If you are interested in a healthy eugeria, note that the desirable proportions of fatty acids in a well-balanced diet—should be no more than 30 percent of calories consumed from fat. For optimum health, this should be broken down as follows:

Saturated fat   20%
Monounsaturated fat   60%
Polyunsaturated fat   20%

In polyunsaturated fats, the proportion of omega-3 to omega-6 is generally: 1:1.

Adipose Tissue

While fats are absorbed in the intestine as fatty acids and glycerol, our bodies do not necessarily use them immediately. When we do not use them, they are synthesized by the liver into human fat and stored in places we rarely appreciate! Still, the fats we consume are not all that ends up on our stomachs and buttocks. Remember

Table 5.3 Some Oils and Their Composition

	Saturated	Monounsaturated	Polyunsaturated
Sunflower	12%	27%	61%
Soy	15	25	60
Corn	13	30	57
Olive	15	73	12
Rape seed oil	8	62	30
Peanut (African)	20	64	16
Peanut (American)	20	44	36

that excess carbohydrates and proteins also convert into fat, so you should monitor your intake of calories from all the food groups.

Triglycerides
The fatty acids associated with glycerol form the triglycerides. The adipose tissue is the reservoir of triglycerides. They are liberated in the plasma as free fatty acids that can directly be burnt by all tissues, giving them energy when the need appears (in fasting, cold). The hormone that releases the fatty acids is adrenaline, the stress hormone. The hormone that stocks them is insulin. The liver can also transform the fatty acids in acetone, which is eliminated in the urine. The acetone is produced in abundance by obese people on a strict diet. The level of triglycerides in your blood should not exceed 1 to 1.5 g per liter, otherwise you risk hypertriglyceridaemias. In most cases, patients with an excess of fat in their blood display a combination of hypertriglyceridaemia and hypercholesterolaemia. Mostly, hypertriglyceridaemia is the result of overindulgence in alcohol or rich foods, but, in a few cases, the condition originates in their bodies. In other words, on occasion, we can put the blame on our genes. A well known study, the "Paris Study," monitored 7,000 men and showed that hypertriglyceridaemia can cause death by itself, without high cholesterol as a contributing factor. Of the 7,000, some subjects died with normal cholesterol levels.

Cholesterol

No doctor denies cholesterol's bad reputation. And this has to do with its obvious contribution to the formation (sometimes with calcium salts) of the notorious atheromatous plaque ("artery goo"), which silts up and obstructs our precious arteries. Though cholesterol can build up in every artery, it is particularly dangerous in the small coronary arteries that supply blood to the heart. There, total restriction results in one thing: "Infarction," or heart attack. During infarction, particular parts of the heart are blocked off from the blood supply and are disastrously damaged. At worst, the damage is so severe, that your heart stops beating. If you don't die, you must live with a significantly weakened heart and will need to follow a program of treatment, surgery, rehabilitation, and therapy for it to heal. No doubt it is in our best interests to take as many preventive measures as possible to avoid coronary attack. It's a gloomy scenario, but once you have had one attack, you will be at risk for another for the rest of your life. Therefore, if you don't willingly monitor your cholesterol, the health of your heart, and diet and lifestyle, you might be forced to do so under quite stressful circumstances. Do as much as you can to avoid an attack. Commit to a healthy eugeria, and as soon as you can.

Predicting Heart Attack
We used to believe that by simply measuring our cholesterol levels, we could then measure the risk of attack. At levels exceeding 1.40 to 2.40 g per liter, we thought the cholesterol would deposit itself in the artery wall, where it would decrease its caliber and therefore its efficiency. Nowadays, we know more: As it is insoluble in water, cholesterol binds with large protein molecules to form lipoproteins, compounds that actually transport cholesterol. These lipoproteins are classified into two groups and have opposing properties.

LDL *and* HDL

First, low-density lipoproteins (LDL) form the villainous athero-matous plaque and facilitate the deposit of cholesterol in the ar-teries. On the other hand, high-density lipoproteins (HDL) play a protective role. They capture the excess cholesterol and deliver it to the liver, where it is metabolized and eliminated. Even if you are healthy, you should be careful to measure cholesterol lev-els at least once a year. Usually, the procedure measures your to-tal cholesterol levels as well as the corresponding HDL levels. Your risk for heart attack is measured according to the high per-centage of LDL levels against low HDL levels. If your cholesterol levels are high, then you should discuss treatment approaches with your doctor and schedule more frequent testing. Many studies, involving hundreds of thousands of people (including the famous Framingham study I mentioned earlier) have researched the var-ious risk factors involved in cardiovascular diseases. Every single study demonstrated that high cholesterol was the most significant contributing factor. Other studies prove that by lowering total cholesterol levels, and by controlling the proportion of LDL to HDL, then the buildup of plaque is retarded and possibly de-creased. Therefore the risk of attack is actually diminished.

To quote a well-known French authority, Professor De Gennes: "With cholesterol levels of 240 mg/dl to 270 mg/dl, many people are treated unnecessarily. Where levels of 200 mg/dl to 250 mg/dl are present, doctors should study the entire fat profile. If the pro-file is normal, there is no reason to treat. But if the total choles-terol level reads 200 mg/dl and a very low HDL level is present, then the patient must be treated."

Homocysteine

I must remind you that high cholesterol is not the only factor con-tributing to atherosclerosis. Recently, scientists discovered that ex-cess levels of an amino acid called *homocysteine*, when it becomes oxidized, can result in clogged arteries that lead to heart disease. A particular study revealed that 25 percent of those with clogged arteries in the heart, 50 percent of those with clogged arteries of the brain, and 65 percent of those with clogged arteries in the lower limbs actually display normal or even low cholesterol. It is possible that homocysteine is the cause of their problems, but there is still much research to be done in this area. There is even some debate over what is considered normal levels at all. Before you get too depressed about this, I will explain how excess homocysteine can be treated successfully with vitamins B_6, B_9, and B_{12}.

Cholesterol, Free Radicals, and Antioxidants
In 1985, two American scientists, Michael S. Brown and Joseph L. Goldstein won the Nobel Prize for Physiology and Medicine, for their discoveries concerning the regulation of cholestrerol metabolism, by demonstrating that when LDL is oxidized, it produces free radicals. Further, the free radicals produced by LDL are absorbed by cells called *phagocytes*, which capture and digest foreign bodies, such as other cells or bacteria. Filled with fatty matter, the phagocytes transform into spumous cells which stick to the arterial wall and begin the development of atheromatous plaque. Once this process was discovered, doctors developed a breakthrough new treatment for high cholesterol. They simply inhibited the early stages of high cholesterol by introducing antioxidants into the system. In other words, they took steps to prevent LDL from oxidizing.

Sources of Cholesterol
At least one-third of our cholesterol comes in our food. The other two-thirds is produced in our liver, where cholesterol is also broken down and eliminated. One enzyme, the tongue-twisting HMG CoA reductase, is responsible for regulating our congenital production of cholesterol. Quite simply, if we inhibit this enzyme, we

inhibit cholesterol production. As soon as scientists discovered this, a new class of drugs—known as *statines*—appeared on the market, to aid this inhibition.

Cholesterol Derived from Food
To monitor our cholesterol levels, we must first monitor the quantity and quality of the fats we ingest and our overall caloric intake. In a word, don't overeat! The bottom line is this: Foods rich in cholesterol and saturated fatty acids favor high cholesterol. And foods containing polyunsaturated fats decrease it.

Recommendations for Cooking
Since most animal fats are made of saturated fatty acids, I suggest you cook with oils that are rich in monounsaturated fatty acids like olive oil, as well as oils containing polyunsaturated fatty acids like corn and sunflower oil. Mind you, polyunsaturated oils have come into disrepute recently: Some nutritionists claim that under oxidation, these oils produce excessive free radicals, though they also contain free radical fighting vitamin E. Unfortunately, this inherent vitamin E is most often consumed by the oil's own free radicals, and that is all it can do as an antioxidant. Remember, the total fat consumed by older people on a daily basis should not exceed 45 g. Some nutritionists suggest you eat even less (see Table 5.4). Roy Walford, who subscribes to a lower calorie intake than most recommends 30 grams, as does Barry Sears, author of the currently popular "Zone" diet.

Table 5.4 Percentage of Fat in Animal Products

Red meats	15 to 20%.
Poultry	10%
Fish	2 to 13%

Cholesterol in Foods

Certain foods are particularly high in cholesterol, for example, one egg contains 240 mg. In fact, an egg can raise the cholesterol level in your blood by 10 percent. Table 5.5 shows percentages of cholesterol per 100 g of various foods.

What to Do about Cholesterol?

Suppose your cholesterol level is high, say at 4 g per liter. If you embark on a calorie-restricted diet that limits the intake of saturated fats and cholesterol, and you include sufficient mono- and polyunsaturated oils, you could reduce your cholesterol by 15 or 20 percent in a month. However, do not assume that this makes you safe. You should know that your problem probably includes a genetic component, and you may need further treatment with drugs to reduce your cholesterol to an acceptable level.

Table 5.5 Percentage of Cholesterol in Various Foods (per 100 g)

Egg yolk	1,560 mg
Kidney, liver, brains, sweetbreads (in decreasing order)	400 to 280 mg
Crustaceans	
Lobster	208 mg
Shrimp	140 mg
Meat	
Beef, pork, veal, mutton (in decreasing order):	120 to 70 mg
Poultry	
Chicken, turkey, chicken liver:	90 to 200 mg
Fatty Fish	
Herring, mackerel, tuna, salmon:	60 to 80 mg
Dairy	
Low-fat milk, whole milk, half and half, cream, cheese, butter (in increasing order)	14 to 280 mg

Diet and Exercise

Do not slack on exercise, because being sedentary, especially in warm weather, decreases your expenditure of calories and increases your fat reserves. Quite simply, we use up more energy when we move or are cold. On the other hand, when you commit to a healthful, calorie-conscious diet and an appropriate exercise program, you use up excess energy, reduce fat reserves, and strengthen your heart and the arteries that supply it with blood.

The result is a more efficient supply of blood to the whole body. Also, not only will you reduce your risk of heart attack, but where infarction occurs, the severity of the attack will be greatly reduced.

Genetic Factors that Contribute to High Cholesterol

Hereditary Hypercholesterolaemia   Hereditary hypercholesterolaemia depends on the inheritance of a particular gene, and is identified by telltale deposits of cholesterol—known as *xanthomas*—under the skin and around the joints. Hereditary high cholesterol is rare but extremely dangerous. Therefore, physicians have developed a program of genetic substitution, whereby they manipulate a patient's genetic structure to address the problem. In fact, most diagnoses of high cholesterol involve a variety of factors, including diet, lifestyle, and several genes involved in the metabolism of lipoproteins.

Stress and Anxiety   The stress of everyday life is a factor contributing to hypercholesterolaemia. Quite simply, stress increases your production of adrenaline, the hormone that mobilizes your fat reserves, which in turn increase fat in the blood. If you live in a big city, know that you are particularly prone to nervous exhaustion.

Low Cholesterol

You might think that the best cure for hypercholesterolaemia is no cholesterol at all. Surprisingly, this is far from the case. A diet extremely low in fats—added to a genetic propensity—can cause low cholesterol and that is a health hazard, especially for older people. While it is clear that high cholesterol levels contribute to the overall risk of mortality, doctors have also identified an increased risk of death by low cholesterol (hypocholesterolaemia). With low cholesterol, there is often a corresponding presence of cancer. A group of women with an average age of eighty-two were observed over a period of five years.

Researchers found their mortality rate was three times higher with hypocholesterolaemia than if they had high cholesterol. Most deaths were due to infectious diseases. The bottom line? Low cholesterol contributes to lowered immunity. In this particular study, the lowest mortality appeared where cholesterol levels stabilized at around 2.7 g per liter. I believe, in eugeria, raised cholesterol levels may well be a phenomenon of adapting to aging. In fact, these increases serve to maintain our cell membranes as well as to strengthen our aging immune systems.

If you have lived with high cholesterol all your life yet have watched your diet, exercised, and even controlled it with drugs and your cholesterol level measures below 3 g per liter. And, having done all this, you turned seventy without ever having a heart attack or stroke, then you can pat yourself on the back! In eugeria, not only are you successfully staving off heart attack, but you are less likely than others to die of deadly infection or cancer. But I do not mean you should let your guard down. Always remain vigilant and continue to monitor and reduce your risk factors: High blood pressure, smoking, drinking, obesity, diabetes, and stress.

And if, at age seventy, you measure low cholesterol, eat more eggs, shrimp and lobster. Why not reach for the caviar! Though medical authorities do not provide guarantees, this may be a way to boost your resistance to cancer and diseases. Unfortunately, research into the effects and treatment of low cholesterol are rare, and not yet definitive. I liken our current knowledge to our knowledge of alcohol. While it is becoming increasingly apparent that a little alcohol each day is a health benefit, we are more likely to condemn alcohol because excess—not to mention addiction—is extremely dangerous. High cholesterol defies a healthy eugeria, a reasonable amount supports your good health, and low cholesterol can compromise your well-being. Reduce your cholesterol, but do not try to rid yourself of it all. Anything beyond normal is a threat to your health, and for a healthy eugeria, my prescription is this: Talk to your doctor. And submit to medication or lifestyle changes if he or she recommends it.

SIMONE

All these risk factor related to nutrition and food components certainly need to be studied to modify your diet accordingly. This is a difficult thing to do as it calls on us to change our bad eating habits. I have experienced it with the good doctor and his health problems.

Dear, I am not revealing a great secret if I tell our readers that you always had a problem with high lipids and cholesterol and also a high uric acid that culminated sometimes in gout attacks if you didn't take your medication or indulged in some fancy foods such as offal or crustaceans.

I have always considered myself the guardian of your good health, and I must admit that you were very cooperative at home, accepting the simple, fat-free diet that I had the cook prepare for you.

But the problem was when we ate out at friends, or with friends in a restaurant, and I insisted that you stick to your diet.

Me: "Darling, don't eat this excellent foie gras, just help yourself to the endives."

Our hostess: "Please, Simone, just for once, it won't hurt him."

Me: "Once today! But tomorrow we have another dinner, and so on. It's bad for him, it's forbidden today, and tomorrow. I know him; he is so weak in the presence of good food that he will not resist if I do not intervene."

This is how I acquired, among our friends, the reputation of being so authoritative with my beloved husband.

My only answer: "When I will be tired of him, I will feed him all these excellent rich foods."

Be prepared to be treated the same way if you live with someone who must absolutely follow a strict diet and try to help.

I have read in advance all the way through the next chapter on the risk factors related to the deficiency of minerals, trace elements, and, vitamins ending up in a list of different items to review:

- *their chemical nature*
- *their activity, the symptoms of a deficiency*
- *where they are found*
- *the recommended daily allowance* (RDA)
- *their use as supplements*
- *the side effects*

I have a suggestion: Let the reader go quickly through this chapter and then come back to it later if he or she wants more precise information on a special vitamin or mineral.

I make this suggestion since we are all anxious to get to the next (more practical) chapter where you give us your recommendations and treatments for eugeria.

CHAPTER SIX

Minerals, Trace Elements, and Vitamins

Sodium chloride is the main component of both human fluids and seawater. Why? Because in the beginning, all life emerged from the oceans. We are the offspring of both sea and earth, and our bodies require a number of minerals to function effectively. We normally ingest all the minerals we need with our food, then eliminate what we don't need in our urine, stools, and sweat. However, certain diseases or treatments can disturb the cycle of absorption and elimination, which in turn disrupts our metabolism.

MINERALS

Sodium, Potassium, Chlorine

Sodium

Sodium, potassium, and chlorine maintain the balance of fluids in our bodies. For this reason, they are fundamental to life. Sodium occurs in different salts, namely bicarbonates, phosphates, and, most of all, chlorides. The most common of all is sodium chloride—that is, table salt! If you live in a temperate climate and expend a moderate amount of energy, all you need is 6 g per day. If you live in a hot climate, or you exercise frequently, you probably excrete more salt through your sweat, and you need more. In extreme conditions, fluid-containing water, salt, and urea can be lost to the tune of fifteen liters per day. At worst, this translates into a loss of 15 to 20 g of salt, which you must replace. If not, you will experience a sodium deficiency (known as *hyponatremia*) and suffer the symptoms of tiredness, nausea, and loss of appetite. In our modern world, however, we are more likely to eat too much salt, and most doctors and nutritionists advise us to cut back. Excess salt intake is dangerous. It leads to the risk of heart and kidney failure, as well as high blood pressure.

Potassium

While sodium collects in the fluids between our cells, potassium concentrates inside them. This mineral is otherwise known as *kalium*, or by its chemical symbol *K*. Its job is to maintain a precise balance of the fluid in our cells, but it also helps to regulate our heartbeat, the contraction of our muscles, and our nerve impulses. Ideally, the level of potassium in our blood (measured as kaliaemia) is maintained around 4 mg per liter, and our daily need for the mineral ranges between 800 to 1,300 g. If you eat potatoes, squash, spinach, legumes, watermelons, oranges, brussels sprouts, bananas, or yogurt, you probably receive more than enough! It is difficult to end up with a potassium deficiency, especially if you eat a variety of healthful foods. Nevertheless, certain conditions (such as diarrhea) and certain medications (such as diuretics) can create problems. Then your doctor may prescribe a potassium supplement. Too much potassium—more often than not the fault of over supplementation—can cause diarrhea, nausea, stomach pain, and vomiting. Less common, but equally worrying, is confusion, irregular or slow heartbeat, numbness, shortness of breath, unexplained anxiety, or unusual fatigue and muscle weakness.

Chlorine

Chlorine is known for its mobility. Chlorhydric acid, born of chlorine, is part of the gastric juices, which digest our food and bring the broken-down nutrients to our cells. There is a reason for chlorine's mobility: It passes through cell membranes quickly and easily. In the plasma, that is the fluid part of our blood, chlorine combines with sodium to form sodium chloride (ClNa), the common salt we already discussed. When chlorine withdraws from our blood, the remaining sodium combines with oxygen and hydrogen to form a sodium base (NaOH) that neutralizes excessive acid inside us. Alkaline bicarbonates and phosphates also form a buffer system to maintain the acid base balance of the blood. This is the pH, which is normally 7.4. A balanced pH is of vital importance. Although it is important for us to appreciate our need for chlorine, there is little need for you to wonder if you are getting enough. It is safe to assume you receive plenty by the salt that is added to so many processed foods.

Calcium

However, do not assume you receive enough calcium. This particular mineral is essential to your health, especially if you are an older woman. It gives our bones and skeletons their rigidity. In adults, the calcium in the skeleton reaches around 800 g—that is 99 percent—of the total quantity of calcium in the entire body. Still, calcium levels in the bones are not stable.

Scientists have discovered that there are constant exchanges between our bones and blood, in order for the level of calcium in the blood to remain stable—around 100 mg per liter. Therefore, when there are depleted levels of calcium in the blood, then our bodies draw calcium away from our bones. Conversely, when we have more than enough calcium in our blood, then the excess is stored in our bones.

A minor amount of 85 to 115 mg of calcium per liter of blood is enough to control the functioning of our muscles and nervous system. It follows, therefore, that a calcium deficiency causes abnormal excitability in our muscles and nerves, which may result in convulsions, tetany, and spasmophilia—unpleasant disorders associated with severe muscle spasm.

Along with vitamin K, calcium is also necessary to coagulate blood. The parathyroids, two small endocrine glands located just behind the thyroid gland, are responsible—along with vitamins D and K—for regulating the metabolism of calcium in our bodies. What is more, calcium can only be absorbed in an acid environment, that is, in the duodenum at the end of the stomach, and only with the help of biliary salts and vitamin D.

If you are fond of rhubarb and sorrel, you should know that these foods contain oxalic acid, which can inhibit the absorption of calcium, as can a substance called *phytin*, contained in the husks of cereal grains. Also, phosphorous affects the absorption of calcium, depending on the ratio of calcium to phosphorous in the food you eat. Just so you know, the ideal ratio for adults is 0.7 calcium to 0.5 phosphorus.

Calcium is most commonly found in milk and dairy products. One quart of milk contains a whopping 1,200 mg. If drinking milk or eating other low-fat milk products does not appeal to you, then make sure you eat plenty of leafy green vegetables such as broccoli, sardines, salmon, or tofu.

I recommend you eat a daily average of 800 mg of elemental calcium if you are male, and 1,500 mg if you are a woman over fifty years old. This means you probably need to include calcium supplements in your diet, besides selecting calcium-rich foods. When choosing a supplement, be sure the milligrams quoted on the label refers to the amount of elemental calcium, not the strength of each tablet. Further, I do not recommend you choose bone meal or dolomite supplements as a source of this mineral, as both have been found to contain unhealthy amounts of lead, an insidious toxin. Also, be sure to take your calcium supplements an hour or two after your meals, for more effective absorption. And be careful that you select a calcium supplement that is easily dissolved. Some disintegrate too slowly to be digested. Play it safe: Buy products that feature the USP logo. I repeat: Supplementation is essential for a healthy eugeria. These are the years when you must concern yourself with osteoporosis and avoidable fractures. Many older people do not get enough sun, or they lack organic lactase to digest milk products and extract calcium from them. Except in the case of spine fractures, recent studies show that calcium—together with vitamin D—significantly decreases the incidence of fractures in older people. More recent studies even suggest that calcium helps lower problematic high blood pressure. There is no good reason not to take calcium. In terms of side effects, few have been identified. Sometimes, and only when the mineral is injected intravenously, do people flush or experience the sensation of heat rushing through their bodies. At worst, expect constipation, a dry mouth, increased thirst, or a metallic taste in your mouth as the minor side effects of taking too much.

Phosphorus

Remember that we measure phosphorus in relationship to calcium. And a healthy ratio of calcium over phosphorus measures at half or slightly higher. Phosphorus complements calcium, most notably in our bones. There, phosphorus levels hover at 450 g—as much as 99 percent of the total phosphorus in our entire bodies. However, the remaining 1 percent is also important. It helps create the essential molecules in the nucleus of our cells, as well as cell membranes. Moreover, our nervous tissue is especially rich in phosphorus. This is because nervous tissue is bound by fat which, combined with phosphorus, creates essential phospholipids abundant in brain cells.

Yes, phosphorus is brain food! You receive it in fish, meat, poultry, meat products, eggs, legumes, and nuts. Lecithin extracted from egg yolks and soy is particularly rich in this mineral. In fact, in these products it is already in the form of a phospholipid.

Our daily need for phosphorus runs at 800 mg. A normal diet produces enough. Therefore, in eugeria, you do not need to supplement, especially as there are numerous contraindications associated with overdose. For one thing, excess phosphorus inhibits the effect of many drugs, such as anti-inflammatories, antihypertensives, antacids, and cortisone. Otherwise, expect confusion, convulsion, muscle cramps, irregular heartbeat, or shortness of breath if you are exposed to too much.

Magnesium

Magnesium is essential to the balance of different ions (minerals) in our bodies, and it also plays a role in the workings of numerous enzymes. Magnesium decreases the excitability of the neurons in our nervous system, and by doing so, it helps trigger healthy muscle movement as well as a steady heartbeat. Half of all the magnesium in our bodies penetrates our bones. We usually carry 20 mg per liter of blood. However, a deficiency precipitates an instant decline, and an immediate increase of neuromuscular excitability. This appears clinically as tremors, muscle spasms, and an irregular heart rhythm.

Look for magnesium in unpolished whole grains, leafy green vegetables, meat, milk, nuts, bananas, and apricots. Our daily requirements are 350 mg for men and 280 mg for women. A deficiency in magnesium can be innate, due to a congenital anomaly, usually to do with our individual metabolism. Otherwise, it is caused by insufficient intake (generally triggered by malnutrition or alcoholism), unsuccessful digestion (brought on by chronic diarrhea, a compromised intestinal transit due to bowel resection or fistulas), or excessive excretion by the kidneys (often brought on by diuretics).

In older people, blood levels of magnesium are generally lower than the rest of the population. That is why many older people battle night cramps. Fortunately, a magnesium supplement can help ease those cramps fairly quickly! And since magnesium is also essential to the efficacy of the different vitamins, there is no justifiable reason not to take a supplement.

The first 100 mg are generally supplied by a good multivitamin, multimineral. The amount in your "multi" may well be sufficient, but I see no reason why you should not take an additional supplement of calcium and magnesium. I have looked at many multivitamin, multimineral supplements, and few of them supply enough magnesium or calcium. I take a supplement that includes 133 mg magnesium oxide, and 333 mg calcium carbonate. That amounts to three tablets a day, so I cover myself with 400 mg of magnesium and 1,000 mg of calcium daily.

Here is an odd warning: Never submit to a combined magnesium and calcium shot, because taken together—in this form—their association is less effective. However, this is not the case in combination oral supplements: In this form they are absorbed without any problem. Side effects of magnesium are minor, but watch for stomachaches and diarrhea. Do not worry unnecessarily: Most supplements are coated to protect the stomach.

Sulfur

Sulfur is part of many proteins. It is found in meat, fish, soy, cereals, vegetables, and peanuts. It is also found in insulin and vitamin B_1 (thiamin). Our bodies contain approximately 100 g of sulfur and our daily needs for it extend to 5 g. There is no question that normal nutrition supplies us with plenty of sulfur, and therefore no supplementation is necessary.

Iron

Iron is an indispensable metallic element. Its main job is to help create the hemoglobin molecule, which is responsible for giving blood its red color and for transporting oxygen to our organs. Iron is also part of myoglobin molecules, which, specifically, supply oxygen to our muscles.

Our adult bodies contain approximately 5 g of iron. One-half exists in the hemoglobin, and the balance is stocked in our spleen and liver. Doctors call this the "martial function" of these particular organs.

Iron is also part of certain enzymes and proteins. In the same way that calcium is absorbed only in an acid environment, an insufficient acid level in the stomach, along with excess phosphorus, inhibits the absorption of this basic mineral. It follows then that if you ingest vitamin C with your iron, it is more easily absorbed into your body.

You ingest iron when you eat lean red meat, poultry, fish, legumes, nuts, dried fruit, and some vegetables. Since many kitchen utensils are made of iron, it will come as no surprise to you that cooking in iron pots also adds iron to your food! The official recommended daily allowance is 10 mg of iron per day for men after fifty-one years. I advise women to take 10 mg after their fifty-first birthday, or after menopause, whichever comes first.

Vegetarians are most inclined to a deficiency, since most iron is found in meat and meat products. Nevertheless, iron deficiencies are relatively rare, except where a person hemorrhages after an accident.

To my mind, excess iron is more of a problem than any deficiency. Quite simply, too much iron facilitates free radical damage to our cells. What is more, excesses have been reported to increase the risk of heart disease and cancer. That is why I advise against supplements. If you are not prone to anemia, or low iron in your blood, leave well enough alone. Further, when selecting your multivitamin, multimineral supplement, choose one that includes low (below 15 mg) or no iron in it. And if you are not sure about your condition, ask your doctor to check the results of your regular blood tests.

TRACE ELEMENTS

Trace elements are actually minerals and are often grouped with them. While we only need these metalloids (metals) in infinitesimal doses, trace elements are essential to our enzymatic systems. That is why you will find them included in any good multivitamin, multimineral supplement.

Iodine

Very small amounts of iodine (100 to 150 mcg—one thousandth of a mg) are necessary for life due to the participation of this metalloid in the function of the thyroid gland, which regulates our basal metabolism. 40 to 50 mg of iodine are found in our adult bodies. Iodine represents 22 percent of what the thyroid weighs. Iodine originates in seawater and marine vegetables, and you will find that iodine levels in soil vary significantly according to how close you are to the coast. On land far from the sea, where the soil and water (thus the flora and fauna) show poor iodine levels, our food is likely to lack this essential trace element. Such deficiency results in hypothyroidism, and at worst—often in mountainous areas— endemic goiters (an enlarged thyroid) or mental deterioration, ending in cretinism. In a few mountainous countries like Switzerland, the government ensures that iodine is added to table salt so that its citizens ingest what they need—that is a daily amount of 150 mcg.

Certain vegetables—such as cabbage—contain substances that conflict with iodine, to the extent that our thyroid is unable to use it. Despite this, I do not believe supplementation is necessary as long as you eat fish or shellfish on a regular basis. Otherwise, seaweed is rich in iodine: If you like Japanese food, the seaweed in sushi or miso soup will definitely supply you with enough iodine. If you eat neither fish nor sushi, select a multivitamin, multimineral, which includes iodine. I repeat: You don't need much iodine, but you cannot afford to avoid it entirely.

Zinc

Zinc acts like a vitamin and, like iodine, it is also necessary to the proper functioning of many enzymes. In particular, zinc works with copper in an enzyme called *superoxyde-dismutase*, which has the all-important job of capturing free radicals. In addition, this helpful trace element has many important functions: It is indispensable to the action of certain hormones, such as the growth hormone and insulin. It helps our immune system by bolstering the health of the thymus responsible for producing the hormone thymulin. In turn, thymulin produces lymphocytes, which are important immune workers.

Zinc acts as an antioxidant, as it stabilizes our cell membranes. It helps to make sperm. It plays a role in some sensory functions like vision and taste. Need I persuade you further? To ingest enough zinc is almost imperative.

You will find this friendly trace element in shellfish, particularly oysters. I lived in Tahiti for years, and so I enjoyed delicious raw oysters, served with lemon and white wine!

If oysters are too exotic, too expensive, or unavailable to you, try any lean red meat, fish, milk, cereals, or legumes. However, you should know that cereals contain phytates, a compound that hampers our absorption of zinc. The same problem occurs with iron, copper, and alcohol—be aware that these substances will deter your absorption of zinc quite significantly.

We usually have around 2 g of zinc in our adult bodies. And to maintain these inherent levels, I suggest men ingest 15 mg of zinc per day, and women ingest 12 mg. In normally nourished adults, deficiencies are rare, but since zinc is most abundant in animal proteins, I believe vegetarians should be extra watchful of their zinc levels. Often, old age and stress necessitates augmentation. Therefore, for those in eugeria, I recommend supplements of 15 to 30 mg of zinc per day. Further, I advise you to select zinc gluconate over zinc sulfate as it is best tolerated by the aging body. Actually, a new product, zinc monomethionine, is also a good choice, as it furnishes both zinc and methionine, an essential amino acid containing sulfur, which is also a potent antioxidant.

Never take zinc with copper, tetracycline (an antibiotic), phosphorus, or iron. In fact, leave at least two hours between taking zinc and the others because zinc can significantly compromise their efficacy.

There are side effects associated with large doses of zinc, say over 30 mg per day. These include chills, fever, mouth ulcers, heartburn, nausea, and unusual fatigue. Also, surprisingly, while sufficient zinc boosts our immunity, excessive zinc can actually suppress it. For safety's sake, do not take doses higher than 30 mg a day over and above a diet that includes foods rich in zinc. And alternate your supplements. Take your supplement for one month, then take a month off. High doses of zinc sometimes cause a deficiency of copper and increase the risk of heart disease and anemia.

Chromium

A scientist, Gary W. Evans, gave rats a supplement of chromium picolinate (an organic form of chromium), and lengthened their lives by around one year. Evans is famous because his findings were a breakthrough. Not since Roy Walford's—undernutrition without malnutrition—diet had anyone found a way to prolong maximum longevity. After Evans, we discovered that 90 percent of adults were deficient in chromium, and for a simple reason: Chromium is not easily absorbed from a number of nutrients. This trace element is extremely important. It reactivates insulin, which reduces our blood sugar levels. By this action alone, chromium helps to prevent the process of glycation—the excessive production of glucose—which damages proteins. If proteins damaged by glycation accumulate, then we can guarantee to accelerate aging.

There is more: Recent human trials show that by increasing the action of insulin, chromium aids in the treatment of noninsulin-dependent diabetes. Further, it reduces the level of total cholesterol and negative LDL, while it increases the beneficial HDL levels. It even increases muscular mass as compared to fat mass.

One warning: While it may seem far from human experience, a study more recent than Evans's showed that chromium picolinate induced lesions of the chromosomes in the ovaries of

Chinese hamsters. However, later research reveals that these lesions were probably produced by picolinate, because chromium chloride or chromium nicotinate never produced the same effect. As a precaution, I suggest you select other chromium salts over chromium picolinate, which, for some reason, is most abundant on grocery shelves. The truth is, these studies must yet be confirmed, and we all know that chromium promises many advantages. Therefore, I have nothing against our including a pinch of chromium with our supplements of vitamins, minerals, and trace elements. Remember, 90 percent of Americans show a chromium shortage and ingest less than half what the experts advise.

I endorse chromium supplements. Though it is abundant in yeast (thus in yeasty products, such as beer), offals (especially kidneys), oysters, lobster, shrimp, broccoli, bran, and cereal germs, it is difficult to get enough from our food. In fact, if you think bread and cereal products will provide your daily dose, think again. Most chromium is lost from grains in refining. I recommend 50 to 200 mcg chromium per day. If your blood sugar is normal—that is less than 1 g per liter of blood, then feel satisfied with the minimum chromium you receive in your multivitamin, multimineral. Most "multis" include approximately 65 mcg. Otherwise, if you know your blood sugar runs over 1 g, then try chromium supplements of around 200 mcg, and try to select an organic variety. I repeat, avoid chromium picolinate, and opt for chromium nicotinate. Actually, an inorganic variety, chromium chloride is most often the variety found in your multivitamin, multimineral supplement, but in the end, any type of chromium is better than none.

Besides the very tenuous connection to the ovaries of laboratory hamsters, there are no obvious side effects to taking chromium. The optimum dose is 200 mcg, and while any more is unlikely to cause health problems, there is no reason to take more than the recommended dosage. However, if you are diabetic, consult your doctor before taking chromium supplements. Never act on your insulin levels without first informing him or her.

Selenium

We doctors first appreciated the importance of selenium when Keshan's disease—a form of rheumatoid arthritis affecting Chinese infants—was found to be connected to an absence of selenium in local Chinese soil. In adults, selenium deficiency is revealed by fatigue, muscular weakness, and cardiomyopathy, a disorder of the heart muscle that can become fatal if we fail to treat the deficiency.

Selenium acts as a coenzyme of glutathione peroxydase, a scavenger of free radicals, which protects our bodies against inflammation and cancer. It is active in supporting our immune systems (particularly in terms of immune response) and therefore aids in the prevention of heart disease, HIV infection, various viruses, and even anxiety.

If we lack vitamin E and selenium, we risk the degeneration of our livers. Various animal experiments have clearly demonstrated the synergy between selenium and vitamin E, and so, administered simultaneously, they offer greater protection and action against cancer than they do given separately.

Selenium is found in yeast, crustaceans (oysters again!), other seafood, red meat, offals, grains, poultry, eggs, garlic, and a number of vegetables, depending on selenium in the soil where they are grown. We receive approximately 75 mcg of selenium through our food alone. In fact, most of us eat slightly more than we need, which is 70 mcg.

Note that selenium can be toxic in excess: People who took 1 mg a day discovered deformities developed in their nails and they also suffered from a garlicky smelling halitosis! Those who took 5 mg daily displayed nervousness, nail and hair loss, and the same unpleasant breath.

So long as you do not exceed 300 mcg (0.3 mg) daily, I believe it is safe to take selenium as a supplement. The best protection is gained by 150 to 200 mcg.

You generally get small amounts of selenium (around 25 mcg)

in your multivitamin and multimineral. Add to this amount what you get in your antioxidant formula, say 400 mg of vitamin E and at least 150 mcg of selenium plus beta-carotene, vitamin C, and certain flavonoids. Remember, selenium and vitamin E works optimally in synergy.

Copper

Copper plays a role in the formation of our red blood cells, in bone metabolism, and in our immune systems. It acts—with zinc—as a coenzyme in the activity of superoxyde dismutase, a free radical scavenger. Superoxyde dismutase (also known as SOD) is found in the fluid body of our cells. I am aware that many attest to the miraculous role that copper plays in the treatment of arthritis and certain skin conditions, but so far, I must tell you that none of these claims have been scientifically proven. Copper is found in shellfish (yes, oysters), legumes, whole grains, nuts, potatoes, and offals. Our daily needs range between 1. 5 and 3 mg.

If you lack copper, your risk anemia and osteoporosis. There is clearly little need for individual copper supplements, but if, for any reason, you choose to take copper supplements, make sure you never take it with zinc. A number of studies reveals that zinc decreases the absorption of copper in our bodies. At the same time, your multivitamin, multimineral most likely contains the two elements together, and to my mind, this is not a bad thing. Overdose of copper can cause blood in the urine, diarrhea, fainting, headaches, and at worst, coma, and death.

Manganese

Manganese helps our bodies to produce energy. This is because it helps metabolize all the nutrients drawn from carbohydrates, fats, and proteins and also helps in bone construction. Manganese acts as a coenzyme to the superoxyde dismutase (SOD), the free radical scavenger we discussed in terms of copper. In this case, we find SOD in the power stations of our cells. Here, carbohydrates are transformed into energy. Eat whole grains, nuts, and vegetables, fruits, black tea, and cocoa powder to receive manganese.

Our daily needs range between 2 to 5 mg, all of which is available in a multivitamin, multimineral supplement. There is no need to supplement any further, despite the fact that there are few known side effects associated with manganese. At worst, excess can hamper your absorption of iron.

Fluoride

You have seen enough toothpaste commercials to know that this essential trace element contributes to the formation of bones and teeth. And while most commercials are focused on preventing dental cavities in children, for those in eugeria, it is more useful to know that fluoride assists us in our war against osteoporosis. Organically, we receive fluoride in seafood (especially fish bones) and tea. Otherwise, it is found in most commercial toothpaste. Also fluoride is added to the general water supply in America, varying in degree by area.

Our needs range from 1.5 to 4 mg per day. Though it helps combat osteoporosis, there is no need to seek out additional fluoride in eugeria, unless your doctor or dentist prescribes supplementation for a specific condition. For the most part, we receive plenty in our food and water. If you take too much fluoride, you risk blackened teeth, joint pain, kidney problems, and stomach ulcers. Also, do not take calcium supplements or aluminum hydroxide (to soothe the stomach) at the same time as a fluoride supplement, as they are inclined to conflict with each other.

Molybdenum

Finally, the trace element molybdenum forms part of certain enzymes, which are important for an efficient metabolism. It is not unlike chromium in this regard, and a deficiency can lead to a buildup of toxins in some people. Our daily needs of molybdenum are 75 to 250 mcg, and we generally receive plenty if we eat whole grains, liver, legumes, green vegetables, and drink milk. If not, our multimineral, multivitamin contains an average of 160 mcg, which covers all bases.

VITAMINS

A minimum intake of vitamins prevents deficiencies that might cause severe diseases. An optimum intake allows a better functioning of the organism and of the enzymatic systems, and support your healthy eugeria in more ways than you know.

Vitamins are chemical compounds, present in most foods in varying doses. We need them—not only because they are indispensable to life and maintaining our health—but because our bodies cannot create or even store most of them. We must ingest sufficient quantities on a regular basis.

Actually, the group we call vitamins is not accurately named. Only vitamin B_1 legitimately belongs to the "amine" category, from which these chemicals get part of their name. As for the other part, "vital" means essential. Certainly, the molecules called vitamins are vital to health.

Vitamins are organic and are thus vastly different in nature and substance from minerals and trace elements. Conversely, they are close to essential amino acids and essential fatty acids: All three compounds are organic and must be furnished by food. Indeed, the somewhat arbitrary distinction between vitamins and the others is based on little more than the amount needed of each to sustain life.

Optimum amounts of vitamins range from a few micrograms to 100 mg. Vitamins were first discovered at the end of the nineteenth century. From the beginning, they were identified by their action, were quantified in units, and labeled according to letters of the alphabet. Once a chemical formula was established, each was measured by weight and awarded a (tongue-twisting) chemical name. Nowadays, we are inclined to flip back and forth between the traditional and modern system. Vitamins are referred to by letter or chemical name, and measured in International Units (IU), or in milligrams and micrograms.

Vitamin Deficiency

In eugeria, we are interested in how much we need of each vitamin to stave off deficiency, as well as a program for maximum wellness. When we are depleted of any vitamin, our tissues—and vitamin reserves—are affected immediately. Deficiencies can reach such low levels that our enzymatic functions are weakened and finally disappear. At a critical peak, the clinical symptoms of deficiency follow.

You may think that in our developed countries, where food is abundant, it is almost impossible to miss out on your vitamins. Think again: Most of us do get enough, but there are great numbers of people—particularly older people—who often suffer deficiencies. Mostly, the shortfall is due to not eating enough: Poverty; ignorance; lack of incentive (by those living alone); eating disorders such as anorexia, dietary taboos, fads, and dental problems all contribute to a reduced vitamin intake and lay the groundwork for problems.

In advanced age, our digestive systems are weaker. Yours may be under duress: Your body may not absorb enough vitamins because of improper chewing. or your stomach juices or digestive enzymes may be depleted. Indeed, your stomach juices may lose their acidity. What's more, prolonged treatment using antibiotics or alcoholism can cause malabsorption of the vitamins you consume, especially of the B group.

A few of the vitamins are interdependent: When one is reduced, a deficiency of the other is likely to follow. For example, vitamin C converts folic acid (B_9) into folinic acid, B_9's active form. Conversely, a condition called *rickets* is often precipitated by a combination of too little vitamin D and too much beta-carotene. For the most part, any excess of water-soluble vitamins are excreted in our urine and sweat. If you live in a hot climate or exercise enough to sweat abundantly, you may need more than the normal requirements.

Government Requirements

Most nations have established minimal nutritional requirements, though these vary from country to country. In the United States, they are established by the Food and Nutrition Board (FNB) in terms of recommended daily allowances (RDA) or daily value which is determined by the Food and Drug Administration (FDA). You should know, however, that the RDA guidelines are approximate, and correspond to the needs of the general population, not to individuals or aging citizens. Particular bodies, particular needs, and particular circumstances all play a part, and it would not be unusual if your need for a certain vitamin exceeded prescribed guidelines. At the same time, these guidelines are useful, as they let us know what we need to prevent the onset of clinical deficiencies.

When breeding animals that have been given vitamins in high doses, researchers found that their offspring grew faster and were healthier, too. Our lives would be simpler if the government could apply many things we have learned from the animal kingdom to human lives! But it cannot. While animal testing gives us necessary leads, long-term clinical tests on humans are always essential before the government can prescribe a course of action to the whole population. My point is this: While the minimum intake recommended by the FNB is one thing, many doctors prescribe far greater doses than the government guidelines. For the most part, increasing your intake of vitamins means improved health, better performance (mentally and physically), and decreased disease.

United States Pharmacopoeia (USP)

The United States Pharmacopoeia (USP) is a nonprofit, nongovernmental scientific organization that sets legal standards for strength, quality, purity, packaging, and labeling for nutritional supplements dispensed in the United States. These are standards enforced by the Food and Drug Administration. For your protection, check whether your preferred products feature the USP logo on the label. While the USP stamp of approval is relatively new, and some excellent products are still to be labeled, if you are in any doubt as to the quality of the product, find an alternative that features the logo. Further, the USP has published a *Guide to Vitamins and Minerals* (Avon; 1996), which outlines information on the indications, contraindications, side effects, and proper usage of every nutrient. To my mind, the guide is conservative, especially concerning the possible benefits and useful dosage of dietary supplements. But if you are interested in the officially recognized daily recommendations of a wide range of nutrients, the book is a more specialized study than I offer here.

Vitamins are classified according to their solubility: They are either hydrosoluble in water, or liposoluble in fat (see Table 6.1).

FAT-SOLUBLE VITAMINS

Fat-soluble vitamins are stored in our bodies and can therefore accumulate in toxic amounts. Vitamins A and D are particularly dangerous when they are taken in high doses for a prolonged time.

Vitamin A or Retinol

Vitamin A is actually an alcohol called *retinol* and is often found in the combined form of acetate or palmitate. Natural vitamin A is found in animal products, such as cod or shark liver oil, milk, butter, and eggs.

Table 6.1 Solubility Classification of Vitamins

Fat-Soluble Vitamins

A group	Vitamin A, provitamins A (beta-carotene)
D group	Provitamins, sterols, vitamins D_2 and D_3 Vitamin E
K group	Vitamin K_1, K_2, and K_3

Water-Soluble Vitamins

B group	B_1, B_2, B_3 (PP), B_5, B_6, B_8, B_9, B_{12}
Vitamin C	
Vitamin P	

Provitamins Carotenes

Provitamins, the precursors of vitamin A, are widely distributed in plants. Otherwise known as carotenoids, they are responsible for the yellow or orange pigment in most fruits and vegetables. You may have read about beta-carotene, the most common of these: It is one of the few carotenes transformed into vitamin A in the intestine when our blood needs it.

Vitamin A Activity

Though only a few convert to vitamin A, all carotenes are important antioxidants. Eat tomatoes for lycopene, cruciferous vegetables such as cabbage, cauliflower, and broccoli for astaxanthine and canthaxanthine, and corn for zeaxanthine, all of which are useful provitamins. Otherwise, choose red pepper, paprika, carrots, spinach, apricots, and lettuce for beta-carotene. Before 1969, vitamin A was measured in international units (IU), but nowadays it is measured in micrograms also. One mcg of retinol is equivalent to 6 mcg of beta-carotene and 3,330 IU of vitamin A. As carotenoids and vitamin A act as antioxidants, they contribute to our fight against those cancers caused by warmongering free radicals. However, a Finnish study conducted in 1994, which significantly selected heavy smokers as a sample pool, concluded that beta-carotene negatively impacted its subjects. The incidence of lung cancer actually increased! The truth is that myriad other studies support beta-carotene as a cancer preventive, especially when taken with vitamin E and selenium. Personally, I wholeheartedly subscribe to the beneficial effects of beta-carotene. Further, I advise you to consider supplementation with other carotenoids, such as lycopene, lutein, zeaxanthine, and canthaxanthine. Vitamin A has many uses. Nowadays, some derivatives of retinol—retinoic acid or tretinoine—as well as other retinoids (natural or synthetic) are used to treat precancerous lesions and various skin and bladder cancers. Also, retinoic acid appears in many modern skin ointments as an antidote to the sun damage that causes skin aging.

Vitamin A Deficiency
A recent study proposed that 40 to 60 percent of the United States citizenry receives only two-thirds of the RDA guidelines of vitamin A. How disturbing! If you lack vitamin A, you risk dry, scaly skin, night blindness, dry eyes (xerophtalmia), and eye infections that lead to permanent blindness. Since vitamin A plays a part in the transportation of iron from the liver to the blood cells, you also lay yourself open to contracting anemia. Overall, a vitamin A deficiency results in a depressed immune system and, added to the specific conditions above, you become vulnerable to infection and other diseases. Fortunately, if you replenish vitamin A before irreversible lesions occur—say per supplement of beta-carotene—you can cure the ill effects of deficiency almost immediately, as long as it is administered early enough.

Recommendations
According to the FDA, our daily requirement for vitamin A is 1,000 mcg (1 mg) or 3,330 IU. You could safely take daily supplements of 5 to 10,000 IU (3 mg) for a month, although I suggest 3,000 IU (1 mg) is enough for eugeria. However, since

carotenoids convert into vitamin A and act as antioxidants, I recommend you supplement with beta-carotene instead. I prefer beta-carotene as it transforms to vitamin A only when you need it, and it induces few side effects in excess. In association with other antioxidants, I recommend 20 to 30 mg of beta-carotene taken daily, and in the long term.

Side Effects
Vitamin A is not without side effects: At its most benign, beta-carotene causes yellowing of the palms, hands, and soles of your feet. Taken at high doses, over a long period of time, vitamin A is stocked in the liver. Ultimately, these results in fatigue, headaches, nausea, dry skin, itching, pain and swelling of your joints, and an enlarged liver. Thankfully, these symptoms disappear as soon as you quit or reduce your intake.

Vitamin D

Though we must ingest most of our vitamins, vitamin D is unusual: Vitamin D_3 (cholecalciferol) is produced in our bodies, from hydrocholesterol, a precursor of cholesterol. Specifically, vitamin D is synthesized by our skin when we are exposed to the sun.

Vitamin D is a sterol and is peculiar to animals alone. On the other hand, vitamin D_2 (ergocalciferol) is produced by a provitamin called ergosterol and is abundant in cereals, mushrooms, yeast, and algae. It is also derived from rye ergot, a parasitic mushroom that lives on rye plants. Manufacturers extract ergosterol from the mushroom and treat it with ultraviolet radiation for their vitamin D_2 supplements. We receive Vitamin D_3 in fish, fish liver oils, butter, milk, and egg yolks. While humans synthesize D_3 with the sun, fish produce D_3 in the dark of the water. Sufficient exposure to the sun gives us more than two-thirds of our daily requirements, otherwise we ingest this vitamin by eating fish and red meat.

Vitamin D Activity

Vitamin D is intimately connected to our body's absorption of calcium and phosphorus. It also plays a role in the healthy calcification of our bones, as it helps essential minerals attach to them. Indeed, a subtle balance of activity occurs between the absorption of calcium, its level in the blood, its attachment and release from our bones, and finally, its excretion by the kidneys. This intricate process is regulated by vitamin D, along with a hormone released from the parathyroid, a minor gland situated behind the thyroid. Based on animal experiments, studies of human tissue cultures, and our knowledge that certain colon, breast, and prostate cancers are less incidental in temperate climates, different studies point to the efficacy of vitamin D as a preventive measure, or even as a treatment against these cancers. Further, vitamin D is also used for treating psoriasis, the chronic condition of red, flaky skin.

Vitamin D Deficiency

Lack of vitamin D, which is responsible for rickets in children, causes osteomalacia in adults, a painful condition accompanied by demineralization of the bone that sometimes ends in fractures. It also contributes to senile and post-menopause osteoporosis. Clearly, first-phase treatment for these conditions requires exposure to the sun, as well as vitamin D and calcium supplements.

Recommendations

Even when you do not receive vitamin D_3 from the sun or appropriate foods—for example, if you are a vegetarian—then there is every good reason to opt for a supplement. In fact, I encourage everyone over sixty to take vitamin D supplements as a matter of course. Isn't it true that we are less inclined to go out in the sun? Further, as we age, our intestine absorbs our food less efficiently. With impaired function, vitamin D supplements become even more necessary.

The RDA recommends a conservative 400 IU or 10 mcg for

older adults, but some doctors propose as much as 800 units. Most multivitamin supplements include around 400 IU. No doubt this is quite enough for eugeria, especially if you bare your skin to the sun for thirty minutes per day, and include some animal fats in your diet. Whether you live in California or Alaska, you may vary your intake. Mind you, it may balance out: You probably eat more meat (a rich source of vitamin D), and undoubtedly receive less sun in Alaska. Dare I suggest, that in California, the reverse is true?

Whatever you do, factor in the reality that vitamins A and D are generally added to most cereals and milk. A single quart of enriched milk provides 400 IU of vitamin D in one shot! Do not ignore this, and you will avoid overdose.

Side Effects
Like vitamin A, vitamin D is fat soluble and can accumulate in the tissues. This accumulation can lead to high levels of calcium in the blood which, in turn, leads to serious side effects. Constipation, dry mouth, headaches, unquenchable thirst, frequent urination, and nausea are the more benign symptoms. Later, expect bone and muscle pain, calcium deposits in the soft tissues (especially in the lungs and kidneys), and elevated blood pressure. Therefore, never exceed a safe limit—up to 1,000 IU per day.

Vitamin E

Vitamin E is resistant to heat and acids, but it is easily oxidized. It is composed of tocopherols and tocotrienols, fat-soluble oily compounds, of which alphatocopherol is the most active. Ester alphatocopherol acetate is the most stable form of this amber-colored oil and is most commonly used in dietary supplements. Tocopherols exist in plants (in small quantities), and in milk products, margarine, and eggs. Otherwise, polyunsaturated oil extracted from grains is the richest source of this vitamin, as this heat-resistant vitamin protects the oil from becoming rancid. On average, 50 mg of vitamin E appears per 100 ml of polyunsaturated oil, a sufficient amount to prevent oxidation, but there is rarely enough extra to be used by our bodies. In other words, despite the presence of this antioxidant, we cannot expect the vitamin E in polyunsaturated oils to fortify our battle against free radical activity.

Vitamin E Activity
Mainly, vitamin E works as an antioxidant. It halts a chain reaction initiated by free radicals that damages cell membranes and the fats in our blood. Actually, this vitamin becomes slightly reactive after it meets the free radicals but is regenerated by other antioxidants, namely vitamin C and coenzyme Q10. Similarly, an anti-free radical enzyme known as *glutathion peroxydase*, which contains selenium, also functions in synergy with vitamin E. This is why selenium and vitamin E are always associated in antioxidant formulas.

As an antioxidant, vitamin E works against cancer, atherosclerosis, and other cardiovascular diseases. However, it does much more than that: As a platelet anti-agregant, vitamin E helps prevent blood clotting and is currently being used in the treatment and prevention of Alzheimer's disease. Otherwise, it stimulates our immunity and acts as an anti-inflammatory. For this reason and others, doctors use it to treat arthritis, skin aging, acne, cataracts, and brain damage, particularly Parkinson's disease.

Vitamin E Deficiency
The more polyunsaturated fats we eat, the more vitamin E we need. Though the FDA recommends 15 IU or 10 mg of vitamin E per day, very few adults meet this requirement. Studies in the 1960s and 1970s concluded that American adults only consumed around 8 mg vitamin E per day, and as many as two thirds of children revealed a deficiency.

For years, vitamin E has been known as the fertility vitamin. A deficit in animals causes their testicles to degenerate or the females to abort their pregnancies. Chickens produce infertile eggs. If you believe such problems no longer concern you, note that other studies point to muscular dystrophy and problems with the nervous and vascular systems occurring in animals in the face of deficiency.

So far, no such catastrophic results have been isolated in humans. Certainly, a vitamin E deficiency is nothing compared to a vitamin C deficiency—which heralds scurvy—or beriberi afflicting those lacking vitamin B_1.

Recommendations

How much more proof do you need? I advise all older people to take a vitamin E supplement, quite simply in defense against encroaching deficiency. While the FDA recommendation of 15 IU or 10 mg per day may address such deficiency, this is far from enough to activate vitamin E's excellent antioxidant properties. For this reason I recommend anything between 400 and 800 IU per day, depending on the state of your health, and specifically your state of oxidative stress: You will need more if you smoke, drink, suffer high cholesterol, or are a victim of high pollution and stress. As much as 800 IU is safe, though higher doses have revealed no side effects. Many supplement producers use synthetic vitamin E in their preparations. However, scientists recently discovered that we most easily absorb the natural form of vitamin E, and reject all but the tocopherols closest to our own bodies. In the end, we only use around an eighth of our supplements. Therefore, look for products composed entirely of natural vitamin E or introduce more wheat germ, wheat germ oil, corn, corn oil, almonds, peanuts, and cereals into your diet.

Side Effects

Paraffin oil (for constipation) or cholestyramin (an anticholesterol medication) inhibits the absorption of vitamin E. Similarly, iron and copper supplements somehow interfere with vitamin E's metabolism. Finally, because it is a platelet anti-aggregant, remember to avoid high doses of vitamin E for a few days before surgery.

Vitamin K

What we call *vitamin K* is actually a catchall description for a group of compounds that contain quinones (namely phylloquinone and menaquinone), all of which prevent us from hemorrhaging. Researchers first found vitamin K_1 in alfalfa, then discovered it was present in almost every green plant. Not surprisingly, spinach, green cabbage, and broccoli are the richest sources of vitamin K_1, though you will also find it in margarine and vegetable oils, especially soy. Milk and liver are two of the few animal sources.

Vitamin K_2 is produced in our intestines with the help of certain bacteria. Vitamin K_3, a synthetically produced form of vitamin K, is most common in supplements and in treatments for certain diseases. All three K vitamins behave in a similar way, but K_3, although it is manmade, is actually the most potent of the three. Still, it converts to K_2 in our bodies.

Vitamin K Activity
Recently, researchers discovered that vitamin K helps to calcify our teeth and bones. Previously, most doctors believed the essential function of vitamin K was to bind with calcium for blood coagulation, without which our wounds, minor or otherwise, would never stop bleeding.

Vitamin K Deficiency
Certainly, vitamin K deficiency is the root of multiple hemorrhages, which lead to unpleasant hematomas (blood collected in the tissues) and internal bleeding. Be sure to report any warning signs of blood in your urine or stools to your doctor immediately.

Truthfully, vitamin K deficiencies are rarely a problem. But if you suffer any intestinal disease, jaundice, or obstruction of the biliary ducts, a deficiency may be due to straight malabsorption. In eugeria, we need vitamin K for the healthy fixation of calcium on our bones: It is essential in our battle against osteoporosis and other diseases in which calcium is a factor.

Recommendations

The FDA recommends 70 to 80 mcg per day for most adults. Eat plenty of green vegetables and dairy products, and you will easily receive your daily requirement. As it is fat soluble, vitamin K is readily absorbed with fatty foods, so long as your digestive juices are in good working order. Ultimately, a multivitamin, multimineral supplement will bolster your dietary intake of vitamin K by around 25 mcg. Only consider increasing this dosage if you are treating osteoporosis.

Side Effects

You may be taking anticoagulants for thrombosis or embolism (migrating blood clots that can obstruct arteries). If so, you should be aware that some of the available treatments use coumarin (an extract of rotten hay!), which is antagonistic to vitamin K. At worst, these antivitamins can cause hemorrhages, but can be quickly addressed with therapeutic doses of vitamin K_1.

WATER-SOLUBLE VITAMINS

Vitamin B_1

All B vitamins are water soluble (so is vitamin C). Vitamin B_1 or thiamin was first extracted from the husks of rice in 1910. Soon afterward, scientists found it in high concentrations in brewer's yeast and in the husks and germs of certain cereals. Later, they discovered it in meat, poultry, fish, legumes, and whole meal bread. Vitamin B_1 is composed of carbon and nitrogen. In fact, it is the only vitamin that we can safely describe as an "amine" that contains nitrogen. B_1 also contains sulfur, hence its name, thiamin. The root *thio* means sulfur in Greek. Unhappily, B_1 is lost when cereals are refined, as well as during cooking. Vitamin B_1 does not stand up to heat.

Vitamin B₁ Activity

B_1 is rapidly absorbed by the upper part of the intestine and is transformed in the liver into an active coenzyme called *cocarboxylase*. Primarily, cocarboxylase "burns" carbohydrates, mainly in the mitochondrias—the power center or engine of the cells. At the same time, B_1 helps to metabolize certain amino acids produced by ingested proteins and helps to produce acetylcholine, a neurotransmitter that communicates between our nerves and muscles and participates in memory function. Not surprisingly, Alzheimer's disease is marked by a decrease of acetylcholine in the body, and when thiamin is prescribed in large doses to patients, their memories improve very significantly. A lesser-known but useful characteristic of vitamin B_1 is that it is an excellent insect repellent! If mosquitoes ever bother you in summer, feel free to pop a few thiamin supplements.

Vitamin B_1 works in synergy with the other B vitamins and with magnesium, which helps transform the B vitamins into active coenzymes. For this reason, your supplements should include all the B vitamins in correct proportion (see RDAs), as well as magnesium.

Water-soluble vitamins do not remain in the body for long, so it is prudent to stagger your doses throughout the day. Also, always take them with meals. To prevent and treat brain disease, fat-soluble thiamins allylthiamine and sulbuthiamine are the versions of vitamin B that are absorbed most effectively. Remember, our brain-cell membranes are composed of phospholipids: Water-soluble vitamins may have difficulty permeating them.

Vitamin B₁ Deficiency

Since it metabolizes carbohydrates, a B_1 deficiency causes disorders in your brain, heart, liver, intestine, and muscles where this metabolism occurs. The classical form of vitamin B_1 deficiency is beriberi, first isolated in China in 2600 BC. Beriberi is characterized by the swelling of the legs and feet; neurological dysfunction such as numbness, muscular weakness, and paralysis; and fatal heart failure. Fortunately, modern electrocardiogram tests reveal the onset of lesions in the cardiac muscle before deficiency ends up in tragedy.

Otherwise, minor B_1 deficiency most affects our minds. If you suffer depression, irritability, and memory loss, you may be lacking B_1 in your system. I must stress that insufficient intake or malabsorption of vitamin B_1 is not uncommon in older people. Also, if you eat a lot of raw fish—such as sushi—a fish-borne enzyme known as thiaminase depletes the body of this essential B vitamin. Most commonly, chronic alcoholism is the main cause for deficiency and its related diseases. In treatment, doctors usually prescribe thiamin supplements, specifically in a form called *thiamin chlorhydrate*.

Recommendations
Our requirement of B_1 is about 1.5 mg per day, but if your diet consists mainly of carbohydrates, then you will need more. If your metabolism speeds up by way of fever, hyperthyroidism, or increased exercise, then you should increase your intake as well. Remember that B_1 does not easily survive too much heat.

Side Effects
There are few side effects associated with vitamin B_1. At worst, you might experience an allergic reaction to vitamin B_1 injections, most noticeably difficulty in breathing or an itchy rash on your skin.

Vitamin B_2 or Riboflavin

Vitamin B_2, also called *lactoflavin*, is abundant in milk. It is also found in red meat, cereals, brewers yeast, and eggs, and presents itself as amber crystals. While it is produced in the intestines of many animals, for the most part, we humans must eat our daily requirement of 1.5 mg.

Vitamin B₂ Activity

Vitamin B_2 is essential to growth. It binds with the enzymes that transport hydrogen through our bodies. In its pure form, it is abundant in the retinas of our eyes.

Vitamin B₂ Deficiency

It is vital to our metabolism in myriad ways, but a deficiency does not present us with life-threatening symptoms. The first signs of deficiency are general malaises, combined with bothersome lesions in the mouth and eye membranes. If you experience small sores at the corners of your mouth or tiny red capillaries creeping into your cornea causing impaired vision, you probably suffer a B_2 deficiency. If parts of your stomach have been removed, or you have been treated with certain antibiotics, then you are particularly vulnerable to a deficiency. And under stress, you may require more. In every case, a B complex can help. Not surprisingly, riboflavin is recommended for the treatment of certain eye conditions and is given to patients during eye surgery.

Recommendations

If your health is normal, then you are probably receiving enough riboflavin in your food and multivitamin, multimineral, and there is no need for special supplementation except your vitamin B complex.

Vitamin B₃, Vitamin PP, or Niacin

Vitamin B₃ Activity

Vitamin B_3, a nicotinic amide, has all the properties of a regular B vitamin, but it is also able to dilate blood vessels, and lower cholesterol. Additionally, it assists in transporting hydrogen and repairing our DNA. This means that vitamin B_3 may help protect us against cancer.

It is most abundant in brewer's yeast, but we also receive plenty in almonds, seafood (mainly salmon), and most red meat, especially liver.

Vitamin B$_3$ Deficiency
Loss of vitamin B$_3$ signifies important metabolic dysfunctions that affect your skin, your digestive organs, and your central nervous system, so it's wise to avoid becoming deficient. Vitamin B$_3$ is also known as vitamin PP because it prevents a disease called pellagra. This disease is characterized by three unhappy Ds: Diarrhea, dermatitis and, often, dementia. Doctors treat patients with up to 500 mg of nicotinic acid (niacin) per day, along with vitamins B$_1$ and B$_6$. Regretfully, niacin occurs in many foods in a form that we cannot assimilate. This is particularly true of corn: In Mexico and the southern United States, where corn is a staple, residents often display severe B$_3$ deficiencies. During World War I, thousands of deaths were caused by pellagra. At first, scientists believed the deaths were due to some mysterious infection, then they realized that poverty necessitated an unadulterated corn-based diet for many. Later research showed that local native Americans and native Mexicans treated their corn with lime, and were never stricken with disease. They learned that lime releases B$_3$ in a form we can absorb! You will know tryptophane by the unbeatable sleepiness you experience after eating your Thanksgiving turkey. This is because tryptophane is a precursor of a neurotransmitter called *serotonin* which pacifies us. Internally, tryptophane is also converted into niacin. That is why we use milk to treat pellagra. It contains little niacin, but plenty of tryptophane. Depleted serotonin leads to anxiety, impatience, feelings of frustration, mood fluctuations, sugar cravings, and the tendency to addict to food, tobacco, alcohol, and narcotics. At worst, such disturbed behavior induces violence and suicide. Niacin can help: It can liberate the often scarce tryptophane from its first use as a precursor of vitamin B$_3$ in order to produce serotonin instead. For this reason,

niacin is popular in the treatment of addictive disorders. It is even prescribed to those quitting smoking.

Recommendations
We need 15 to 20 mg of vitamin B_3 per day. There is no need to supplement outside of your multivitamin, multimineral. However, if you suffer high cholesterol, your doctor may prescribe 2 to 3 g of nicotinic acid to treat your disease.

Side Effects
We observe dilation of the blood vessels and flushing of the face with high doses of nicotinic acid.

Vitamin B_5 or Pantothenic Acid

Vitamin B_5, or pantothenic acid helps convert carbohydrates, fats and amino acids into energy in the mitochondrias, or engines of our cells. It converts into coenzyme A in our tissues, the starting point for the production of cholesterol. In turn, cholesterol produces steroid hormones such as cortisone, the sex hormones, DHEA, vitamin D, and coenzyme Q10. Vitamin B_5 helps produce acetycholine, the neurotransmitter that regulates communication between our muscles and nerves and contributes to memory function. A corresponding alcohol to vitamin B_5 is panthenol, which is more easily absorbed than pantothenic acid, though the compound calcium pantothenate is the most stable and less easily destroyed. Look for B_5 in brewer's yeast, offal (kidney and liver), egg yolks, milk, bran, cereals, and vegetables. It is also the major component of royal jelly.

Vitamin B_5 Activity
Vitamin B_5 helps produce cortisone. For this reason, some doctors use it to treat rheumatoid arthritis as well as allergies to pollen

and dust. Pantethin, a biologically active intermediate form of vitamin B_5 lowers high cholesterol and can metabolize alcohol. It is available as a supplement and may be used in the treatment of high cholesterol and alcoholism. As it is important to the creation of energy, and therefore growth, panthenol can be used to treat skin problems and balding, and in doses of 2 g per day many athletes use vitamin B_5 to enhance their performance.

Vitamin B_5 Deficiency
When a group of scientists denied laboratory rats vitamin B_5 for long periods, the animals lost their hair, what was left of it turned white, then they developed sores on their skin. Later, the scientists discovered similar lesions in the rats' digestive tracts, livers, reproductive, and nervous systems. On top of everything else, the poor beasts suffered respiratory disorders, namely runny noses and bronchopneumonia.

After twelve weeks of a diet deficient in vitamin B_5, expect the following symptoms in humans: Headaches, tiredness, numbness, cramps, digestive problems, accelerated heartbeat, sudden slumps in blood pressure (especially when you stand up), insomnia, depression, skin disorders, and balding. Prisoners of war in Asia first revealed a mysterious "burning-foot" syndrome after they were starved of food. Interestingly, their condition was treated successfully by vitamin B_5, yet other B vitamins had no effect.

Recommendations
In the United States, the FDA recommends an intake of 7 mg per day, though the French suggest as much as 3 mg more. Most over-the-counter supplements include at least 10 mg.

In eugeria, extra supplementation of vitamin B_5 is not usually necessary, outside the amount you receive in the multivitamin, multimineral on a daily basis. However, under stress, your body depletes itself of its important resources and you may need more. Take additional vitamin B_5 in a regular B complex, as stress uses up all the B vitamins. Remember, the Bs and magnesium are absorbed best together.

Side Effects
Best of all; don't worry about side effects, as far as my research shows, there do not seem to be any.

Vitamin B$_6$ or Pyridoxine

In small quantities, vitamin B$_6$ is found in animal and vegetable products, especially wheat germ, baker's yeast, bran, liver, fish, nuts, and legumes. Sadly, half of vitamin B$_6$ is lost in refinement and cooking. This vitamin exists in the form of an alcohol, an aldehyde (known as *pyrodoxal*) or an amine (*pyridoxamine*).

Vitamin B$_6$ Activity
Pyridoxine transforms into coenzymes in our bodies, to help us metabolize amino acids and proteins. It also helps create neurotransmitters such as adrenaline, dopamine, serotonin, and GABA; therefore it follows that a deficiency in vitamin B$_6$ affects our nerves and mental reactions. Additionally, vitamin B$_6$ converts tryptophane into vitamin B$_3$.

If you suffer depression, anxiety, convulsions, epilepsy, or carpal tunnel syndrome, your doctor will prescribe high doses of B$_6$, which is useful in treating these particular disorders. Also, this vitamin boosts the immune system and is used to treat cancer, particularly of the bladder.

Vitamin B$_6$ Deficiency
If you are deficient in vitamin B$_6$, expect skin disorders (such as seborrheic dermatitis, a form of acne), lesions of the mucous membranes of the lips and tongue, fatigue, depression, and insomnia.

If you fail to treat your disorder, then expect a depressed immunity, glucose intolerance, and anemia. You may also develop polyneuritis, an unpleasant condition characterized by numbness and weakness of the nerve endings.

Depleted vitamin B_6, along with depleted folic acid (B_9) and vitamin B_{12}, causes significantly high levels of blood homocysteine. In the chapter on fats and cholesterol, you will have read that excessive homocysteine—a type of amino acid—is as dangerous as excess cholesterol, as it clogs our arteries and contributes to heart disease. In fact, our coronary arteries and carotids are the most vulnerable. Unchecked, homocysteine oxidizes, releasing free radicals into our bodies. Further, excess homocysteine also contributes to depression and mental impairment. These are all excellent reasons to get your vitamin B_6.

Recommendations

Often, our regular diet fails our need for this vitamin, particularly if we are older, stressed, or we smoke and drink alcohol. In eugeria, be extra conscientious about taking your multivitamin, multimineral. This way, you can be sure of at least 2 mg of vitamin B_6 per day—which corresponds to the national requirement.

A B complex covers all your vitamin B needs. Select a supplement that includes at least 100 to 150 mg of each, though biotin and vitamin B_{12} are generally included at lower levels, say 100 to 150 mcg per tablet. Also, as an extra precaution, take a calcium-magnesium supplement to ensure the efficacy of the vitamin B_6 you ingest. The optimum approach is to take a B complex for one month, alternating with a brewer's yeast supplement every other month.

Side Effects

There are no serious side effects associated with vitamin B_6 as long as you stick to the prescribed doses. A number of experiments with doses of 50 mg or more, taken over a period of several months, revealed little more than subjects experienced numbness in the hands and feet and became oddly clumsy!

If you take isoniazide, a drug used to treat tuberculosis, note that this drug is an antagonist to pyridoxine. In this case, take higher doses of vitamin B_6, say 40 to 150 mcg more.

Similarly, pyridoxine can inhibit the effect of levodopa—a drug used to treat Parkinson's disease. Quite simply, your best defense is not to take levodopa and vitamin B_6 together.

Vitamin B_8 *or Biotin*

Raw egg whites contain a protein called avidine that suppresses the action of vitamin B_8. After feeding raw egg whites to rats, researchers discovered the protein avidine and, by default, the vitamin biotin of a complex chemical formula.

Vitamin B_8 Activity

As a coenzyme, biotin helps to metabolize carbohydrates and proteins and to produce certain fatty acids. It is found in low concentrations in most animal and vegetable tissues, particularly in yeast, liver, and egg yolks. Also, vitamin B_8 is created internally, by a particular bacteria in our intestine.

Vitamin B_8 Deficiency

Deficiency of vitamin B_8 is rare: That is why scientists first battled to identify what ailed those with the classical symptoms: Fatigue, numbness, lesions on the hands, feet, nails, and hair. Atrophy of the tongue, muscle pain, sleepiness, and depression are also common. Most often, deficiencies appear in alcoholics, as well as from surgical removal of the stomach or treatment with certain antibiotics. Antibiotics, for one thing, are well known to destroy intestinal flora. Either way, you may be unable to absorb biotin.

Recommendations

We need to ingest 30 to 100 mcg of vitamin B_8 per day. Under normal circumstances, there is little need to exceed the 30 mcg or so present in your daily multivitamin, multimineral supplement. However, if you have skin, hair, or nail problems, it is quite safe to take more, if you find that it helps.

Vitamin B$_8$ Side Effects
Even in experiments, when subjects took over 50 mg per day, researchers were unable to pinpoint any side effects.

Vitamin B$_9$ or Folic Acid

Vitamin B$_9$ Activity
Folic acid is extremely important. It aids in the breakdown of certain amino acids: the metabolism of histidine and glycin, the synthesis of serine and methionine, and the production of purine and pyrimidine bases that help create the nucleic acids DNA and RNA. In a word, we need folic acid to produce healthy genes.

Vitamin B$_9$ Deficiency
Though the following statistics are essentially irrelevant to those in eugeria, research reveals that as much as half of all teenagers and women of childbearing age fall dramatically short of enough folic acid. Tell your daughters, granddaughters, and young women friends: In pregnant women, a lack of folic acid increases the risk of neural tube defects such as spina bifida or anencephaly. And these disasters are easily prevented by doses of 400 mcg, as long as they are initiated before and during the first month of pregnancy.

In eugeria, you should know that even a minor deficiency causes tiredness, irritability, mood changes, impaired concentration, and loss of memory. At worst, prolonged deficiency causes megaloblastic anemia, an anemia that features large, immature red blood cells. This condition is also triggered by a vitamin B$_{12}$ deficiency. Chemotherapy causing abdominal pains, nausea, vomiting, and mouth ulcers also signifies a need for B$_9$, as do skin and hair problems.

Further, a shortfall can cause lesions of the peripheral nerves and mental and behavioral disorientation that can end in dementia. Fortunately, mental problems are quickly relieved by a good course of supplements, especially if you catch the deficiency in its early stages.

If you smoke, you will be interested to know that folic acid helps prevent precancerous lesions from developing in the bronchia of your lungs. In addition, vitamin B_9 helps inhibit colon polyps and similar lesions from developing in the cervix of women. Homocysteine—which contributes to atherosclerosis and heart attack—is also associated with low levels of vitamins B_6, B_{12}, and folic acid. However, with sufficient vitamin B_6 in your body, homocysteine converts into cysteine and methionine in the presence of vitamins B_9 and B_{12}.

You may wonder what cysteine and methionine do for you. These two sulfur-containing amino acids have antioxidant properties and, as the joint action of vitamin B_6, B_9, and B_{12} they destroy homocysteine. We trade harmful homocysteine for health-enhancing amino acids instead. In fact, I recommend you take cysteine and methionine as antioxidant supplements on a periodic basis (see the chapter on antioxidants).

Do whatever you can to rid your body of homocysteine. It disturbs the development of your bone matrix. Therefore, it contributes to osteoporosis. It acts as a neurotoxin that is bad for the brain. In fact, it causes brain cells to self-destruct. This leads the way to depression, memory loss, and ultimately, dementia.

Recommendations

Homocysteine is a problem, but folic-acid deficiency causes the problem. Therefore, your first line of defense is to combat the deficiency. Folic acid does more: It helps in a number of diseases in which homocysteine can flourish, though researchers are not yet certain whether folic acid's favorable effect on mental problems is due to its direct action on our brains or to its action on homocysteine. Whichever way you look at it, homocysteine is decreased in the presence of vitamin B_9. And that is a good thing. Make sure you eat green leafy vegetables, yeast, wheat germ, liver, egg yolk, cheese, and red meat. Unfortunately, processing and cooking dramatically reduce the amount of folic acid in food. Why not develop a taste for fresh spinach salad? Ultimately, you should consume at least 200 mcg of vitamin B_9 per day. Most multivitamin, multimineral supplements contain around 400 mcg of vitamin B_9, which is actually sufficient for your eugeria. However, if a blood test reveals high levels of homocysteine, or if you experience cognitive, memory, or cardiovascular problems, this is a clear pointer to include more in your diet. As a precautionary measure, take a B complex as well. Alternate this with brewer's yeast along with a calcium-magnesium supplement.

Side Effects
There are few side effects associated with folic acid. At worst, people who take over 1 mg per day risk an outbreak of hives.

Vitamin B_{12} or Cyanocobalamine

Though its main sources are animal proteins such as red meat and liver, very little vitamin B_{12} is found in food. Like cattle and sheep, we produce cyanocobalamine in our intestine, but the net amount is far from enough. We need to ingest it. This vitamin contains one central atom of cobalt (cyanocobalamine) and is the largest and most complex of all vitamin molecules. Under a microscope, it has the appearance of carmine-red crystals.

To absorb it depends on the "intrinsic factor," a component of our gastric juices. In the presence of calcium, this intrinsic factor unites with vitamin B_{12}, is transferred through the first part of the small intestine and then circulates into our blood. After that, vitamin B_{12} is stored in our liver.

Vitamin B$_{12}$ Activity

Along with folic acid, vitamin B$_{12}$ contributes to our production of blood cells. It also breaks down homocysteine and helps to make methionine and choline, the amino acids that produce neurotransmitters.

Vitamin B$_{12}$ Deficiency

Since vitamin B$_{12}$ is most commonly found in meats, for obvious reasons vegetarians—and older people—are particularly prone to vitamin B$_{12}$ deficiency. Also, atrophic gastritis, a stomach disease common in those over age sixty, causes diminished levels of the intrinsic factor that leads to malabsorption.

Deficiency can also cause macrocytic or "pernicious" anemia, in which red blood cells are retarded in the middle of maturation.

Recommendations

Thankfully, macrocytic anemia is easily treated with vitamins B$_9$ and B$_{12}$. Lesions of the spinal chord and mental deterioration often accompany more advanced cases, as do a distressing number of mental disorders, especially in older people. For this reason alone, I strongly encourage supplementation, since it is so difficult to control our intake of vitamin B$_{12}$, not to mention the levels of homocysteine and methylmalonic acid in our blood. Further, the mysterious and debilitating chronic fatigue syndrome, which has stumped doctors for decades, is now fairly successfully treated with large doses of vitamin B$_{12}$, usually administered by injection. If we lack the intrinsic factor, we can absorb vitamin B$_{12}$ in its crystalline form by way of a supplement. In fact, supplements are a godsend, especially if we cannot absorb vitamin B$_{12}$ with our food. If you are symptom free, your multivitamin, multimineral supplement supplies you with enough vitamin B$_{12}$ in eugeria. Each supplement contains around 6 mcg. Still, as a precaution against homocysteine, remember to take brewer's yeast alternating with a high potency B complex that includes 100 or 150 mg of every

B vitamin except biotin and vitamin B_{12}. These particular Bs usually measure 100 to 150 mcg each.

Vitamin C or Ascorbic Acid

Vitamin C is so close to glucose that many animals actually produce it from glucose. However, as primates, we humans must ingest vitamin C with our food. Most know that vitamin C is abundant in fruit and vegetables, though we also receive it in liver and milk. Less well-known is the fact that vitamin C is the most unstable of all the vitamins. It is easily destroyed by heat, oxidized by air, and dissolved in water.

Vitamin C Activity

Internally, ascorbic acid is transformed into oxalic acid and any excess is flushed out in our urine. That which we need is retained and stored in our white blood cells. We carry vitamin C in high concentration in various organs, particularly in our pituitary gland (which produces our hormones) and our eyes, but we are never able to store it for future use. We excrete the excess almost immediately—hence the orange color of urine indicating we have ingested more than we need! Ascorbic acid helps to oxidize certain amino acids by producing carnitine, an amino acid that helps pump our heart and muscles. Not surprisingly, many athletes take carnitine to enhance their performance. Vitamin C also helps to produce the neurotransmitter noradrenaline and makes collagen, the binding ingredient that holds our bodies together. Calcium is deposited in collagen. It follows then, with a vitamin C deficiency, our body manufactures less collagen, and we become physically weaker. Vitamin C stimulates the cellular defenses of our immune system; thus it guards against infection, particularly viruses. That is why we take vitamin C to avoid common colds. Also, it regenerates vitamin E and glutathione, both potent antioxidants. In fact, as part of an antioxidant defense system, it guards against inflammation, cardiovascular problems, and cancer. During digestion, it prevents nitrates and nitrites (compounds made of nitrogen) from converting to nitrosamine, a degraded chemical compound that can cause cancer.

Vitamin C helps to metabolize iron. Not only is this useful if you are anemic, but it also acts against hemorrhaging and helps to bolster our fragile capillaries. Vitamin C even boosts the activity of our hormone-producing adrenal glands, though no one is sure quite how it does this. In any event—and for this reason—doctors often prescribe it for the postoperative care and during convalescence from many diseases. During infectious diseases, and in all cases of stress, our blood levels of ascorbic acid decrease considerably. Stress and disease also induce us to excrete more. That is why it is prudent to take high doses of vitamin C at such times, for example to treat influenza and colds.

Vitamin C Deficiency

Though most animals manufacture their own vitamin C and rarely display deficiency, we humans have battled a shortage for centuries. On high seas for months at a time, cut off from fresh fruit and vegetables, sailors used to suffer from a disease called *scurvy*. As early as 1750, researchers discovered that lemon juice provided a cure. Then, in 1930, a Hungarian doctor, Szent Györgyi, established that vitamin C was the magic ingredient to fight this disease.

Scurvy begins with weakness, irritability, muscle pains, joint pains and significant weight loss. The first visible signs include bloody, swollen gums and loosening teeth. (Attention toothless older people! Since these particular symptoms may not appear in your case, do not presume you should not take note of the others.) Later, bleeding under the skin, muscular hematomas (pools of blood collected in the muscle), and hemorrhaging in the eyes, stomach, bowels, kidneys, and brain signify scurvy in its advanced stages. Vitamin C is more than a preventive. It is the curative treatment of scurvy, particularly when taken with vitamin P, also abundant in fresh fruit and vegetables, especially lemon juice. Vitamin

P, otherwise known as *citrin*, is a little-known vitamin but it is important. Its main job is to control the permeability of the tiny capillaries that bring blood to our tissues.

Recommendations
Nobel Prize winner Linus Pauling advocated mega doses of ten grams or more of vitamin C per day, though many well-known doctors scoff at his notions, saying such excess leads the way to kidney stones and gout. The truth is, neither Pauling's positive claims, nor the other doctors' disclaimers have been proved or disproved. In any event, there is little question that the vitamin C in your multivitamin, multimineral supplement (around 80 mg) is far from enough. Fortunately, an antioxidant supplement evens out the imbalance: My recommendation is an optimum intake of 500 mg. However, if you drink, smoke, suffer high cholesterol, or are exposed to pollution or lifestyle stress, then there is no reason not to increase your dose even more: Take 1 g per day if you like. That much at least will do you no harm.

Choline and Lecithin

Choline was once regarded as a vitamin—we called it vitamin B_7—but in 1980, it was deprived of this status because scientists suddenly discovered it is produced in our liver! Nevertheless, if ever the production of this amino alcohol falters, or our need for it increases, then we must get our choline in food. Mostly, we get it in lecithin, a phosphatidylcholine, composed of choline, phosphoric acid, glycerol, and fatty acids.

Note that this is not the lecithin added to our foods: Common lecithin is an amalgam of phospholipids, specifically 10 to 20 percent phosphatidylcholine, as well as myoinositol, ethanolamine, and serine. Since it can bind with both water and fats, you will find this form of lecithin in margarine, ice cream, and mayonnaise—it gives these foods their creamy consistency.

Choline Activity

Choline is found in eggs, brewer's yeast, liver, soy, spinach, and cruciferous vegetables, such as cauliflower and cabbage. Phosphatidylcholine is part of practically all our cell membranes but is especially concentrated in our brain tissue. Eat eggs, liver, soy, and peanuts for phosphatidylcholine-rich brain food, which is also transformed by enzymes into choline. In turn, choline combines with phosphates to produce the phospholipids essential to our cell and the health of our brain. Further, choline is synthesized from methionine and serine, which contribute to the production of protein in our body.

Choline combines with acetic acid, acetylcoenzyme A, and vitamin B_5 to produce acetylcholine, a neurotransmitter particularly important to our memory function. In fact, acetylcholine disappears progressively in Alzheimer's disease—another good reason to stock up on choline.

Recommendations

Choline and lecithin (not the food additive) supplements have been prescribed to protect the liver from hepatitis and cirrhosis as well as in the prevention and treatment of liver cancer. In older people, doctors regularly prescribe it as an antidote against cerebral aging. Be sure you select a multivitamin, multimineral supplement in which choline is included, usually in doses of 1.5 g or more. Otherwise, take a lecithin supplement, preferably "softgels" of 500 mg extracted from soy. The best lecithin supplements feature high concentrations of phosphatidyl choline and phosphotidylserine. Make sure you also include calcium and magnesium in your supplement program, since calcium is essential for absorbing phosphorus, and vitamin E compensates for the polyunsaturated fatty acids in soy lecithin.

CHAPTER SEVEN

Risk Factors
Not Directly Related to Nutrition

HIGH BLOOD PRESSURE

High blood pressure is a true risk for heart attack and stroke that must absolutely be treated. Don't worry if your blood pressure increases as you grow older. Within certain parameters, this is perfectly normal. However, you should be aware that our artery walls lose elasticity as we age also. Consequently, if your blood pressure exceeds normal levels, your artery muscles may become dangerously strained. In effect, high blood pressure greatly increases your risk of heart attack. Indeed, the famous Framingham study found that high cholesterol levels were the major risk factor for heart attack in older people; hypertension ran a close second.

Systolic and Diastolic Hypertension

Systolic hypertension (measured when the heart muscle contracts) over 150 cm of mercury is so common that we frequently—and foolishly—fail to take care of it. On the other hand, elevated diastolic blood pressure (when the heart muscle relaxes) is considered more dangerous. We are more conscientious about treating it when it is over 90 or 100.

Two Swedish trials, called *Systolic Hypertension in the Elderly Program* (SHEP) and *Swedish Trial in Old Patients with Hypertension*

(STOP), proved the benefit of treating both forms of hypertension. With care, the incidence of stroke decreased by 36 to 40 percent, and heart attacks were reduced by 27 to 40 percent compared to those who were not treated.

Two-thirds of patients who suffer high blood pressure are between sixty-five and ninety years old, and most suffer systolic hypertension.

Low Blood Pressure

Just because high blood pressure is dangerous, do not assume that low blood pressure ensures optimum health. Far from it. Although drug treatment of hypertension is generally successful, lowering blood pressure does not work for everyone. Some individuals with advanced atherosclerosis must sometimes sustain blood pressure levels higher than normal to maintain the blood supply to their heart and brain.

Lifestyle Adjustments for Minor Cases

Medication is not always necessary to regulate blood pressure. In minor or moderate cases, say 150/100, small lifestyle adjustments should be sufficient. Lose weight, reduce your salt intake, exercise regularly—perhaps increase the length of your workout—and there is an excellent chance your blood pressure will stabilize. In any event, be sure to schedule regular blood pressure checkups and consult your doctor for personalized treatment.

HEREDITY

Heredity certainly plays a role in longevity. Genes can represent higher risk factors, necessitating a reinforced surveillance. Some of us are predisposed to live longer than others and are relatively protected from various diseases related to age. In fact, scientists have already isolated two genes in our chromosomes that affect our life span. They are called APOE and ACE.

Dr. Leonard Hayflick of the University of Philadelphia proved that—on average—a single cell can multiply only fifty times in its life. From this he proposed that our life span is linked to our own genetic clock. Quite simply, we are preprogrammed to die when our time line runs out.

The Issue of Telomeres

The basics of genetics are best explained by analogy: Imagine your entire genetic composition is a library, your chromosomes represent a book in the library, your genes a sentence, and your DNA base a particular character in a single word. Each cell has forty-six chromosomes with two ends identified by their own "telomeres": these are DNA-based aging clocks, which are shortened each time your cells multiply. Remember that we generally die when our cells complete their full cycle of multiplying.

Hope Comes from a Cancer Cell

By studying and manipulating a particular enzyme—the "telomerase" present in immortal cancer cells—scientists are looking at ways to cure this fatal disease. They are also using immortal cell theory in studies concerned with prolonging life. If cancer cells can live forever, then why not the others? This new and complex field of study is best discussed in a book called *Reversing Human Aging*, by Michael Fossel (Morrow 1996.) Though the new research is fascinating, we do not yet have any conclusive results, which are likely a long time in coming. For the time being, we must engage the resources at hand.

A Word about Cloning

In 1997, a humble sheep named Dolly became internationally famous as the first animal ever to be cloned from an adult. While her arrival into our world is exciting, I doubt Dolly will live to a ripe old age. Since the cell that begat her was already mature, Dolly's telomeres have already completed much of their lives—they are as old as her mother's in fact. If Dolly surprises us and lives a normal sheep's life span, then we will have to reconsider the theory of telomeres!

Genes and Disease

Genetic inheritance is undoubtedly a factor predisposing people to various ailments. We have advanced to the point where genes causing some cancers and Alzheimer's are fairly easy to identify, yet, every day, new genes are discovered that point to the onset of less-common diseases.

Cancer

For their capacity to trigger anarchic multiplication of cells in our body, oncogenes are defined by the way they make tumors. These genes are normally activated when we are growing and are supposed to slow down when we mature. Indeed, our bodies produce and store antioncogenes that actually control the multiplication of cells. Unlike oncogenes, our antioncogenes are repressed during the growth period and are activated the moment we reach adulthood. As long as the subtle balance between the activity and nonactivity of these two genes are stable, then you are likely to maintain your good health. However, both oncogenes and antioncogenes can be stimulated into activity by radiation, chemical pollutants—such as tar in cigarettes—or viruses like the papilloma virus causing cervical cancer. When these genes develop unchecked, the result is anarchic—and cancerous—cell growth.

Genetic-based Treatments for Cancer

Despite the surge in our understanding of the genetic origin of many diseases, we have not yet developed any significant treatments. We can only claim to be better equipped to detect your potential for life-threatening illness. If your mother had breast cancer, you can be tested for the gene that causes its development. And, if your doctor establishes that you carry the gene, then you can undergo more frequent mammograms and more vigilant monitoring for the onset of cancer. As always, early detection and early treatment is best.

The Future of Gene Therapy

Most doctors believe that gene therapy will be available in the near future. In fact, a few simple therapies already exist where only one or a few genes are indicated, for example, hereditary high cholesterol. However, genetic therapy for ailments involving a number of genes—such as cancer or Alzheimer's—are still on the drawing board and will be for some time. Exciting breakthroughs are imminent, but let me say this: However great our efforts to enjoy a long and healthy eugeria, we may never be able to escape our heredity. Sadly, biology hardly subscribes to equality or justice: In the end, there is no guarantee we will ever control a particular health crisis fated to befall us.

Still, a number of diseases—which involve many genes—can be influenced by external factors, which we can control. As always, your best defense is a healthy lifestyle. Using all the means and knowledge available, always do what you can to ensure general good health.

IMMUNITY

In every discussion about the immune system, we always identify two different parts. First, our white blood cells (the single nucleus T- and B-cells), and the enemy-devouring "macrophage" polynucleated cells, destroy cells damaged by viruses and defend against tumors. Our white blood cells are so hostile to foreign bodies that they occasionally reject tissue grafts applied during surgery. Second, the humoral (from the body fluids) component of our immune system produces antibodies to fight bacteria and other infections that enter our bodies. Our cellular and humoral immune defenses are connected and interdependent.

Age and Immunity

As we grow older, our immune system weakens. Clinical tests show that 34 percent of older bodies fail to react when injected with antigens that increase our production of antibodies. In most younger people, the antigens cause swelling and redness on the skin. The test indicates the activity of immune defenses in youngsters, but it also reveals weakened immunity in older people.

Why Our Immunity Decreases

A weakened immunity has to do with the normal, age-related atrophy of our thymus gland, which exists to produce disease fighting T-cells. When the thymus gland was removed in laboratory experiments, scientists discovered a sharp decline in the subject's immunity. At the same time, when laboratory animals were injected with the thymus hormone, or old mice were given grafts of thymus fetal tissue, they recorded a significant increase in immunity.

A weakened immunity explains why—despite antibiotics—older men and women are more vulnerable to death by infectious diseases than their younger counterparts. Significantly, 69 percent of these deaths are by complications from influenza—in most cases the flu led to deadly bronchopulmonary infections. Your risk of death by influenza is thirty-five times higher when you are seventy than when you are ten. The second highest risk factor is from urinary infection. And believe it or not, the third highest risk is from a conglomerate of infections that unwell older patients contract in hospitals.

Can Eugeria Help?

A healthy eugeria can boost your immune system.

First, cease any activities that compromise your immune defenses. Quit your use of tobacco and excess alcohol and be mindful of your exposure to harmful radiations, such as X rays. As far as possible, stay out of the sun. UV rays are an anathema to your immunity.

Vitamins

Your multivitamin, multimineral supplement will help. You should take vitamins C, E, and selenium in a robust antioxidant. In addition, increase your intake of vitamin B_6. Vitamin B_6 is vital to a healthy immune system, especially after age forty. The recommended daily dose of vitamin B_6 is 2 mg, though I advise 1 or 2 mg more for extra protection.

Thymus

From the fifties to the late seventies, the use of thymus in a treatment called *Niehans Embryo Cell Therapy* was extremely popular. Cell therapy is out of fashion today. If it was not for ethical reasons, it might reappear in the form of human embryo homografts.

Zinc

Zinc is essential to the health of your thymus gland and therefore aids in the production of your defensive T-cells. The FDA recommends 15 mg of zinc per day, which is usually included in your multivitamin, multimineral supplement. It also occurs in most antioxidant formulas. So long as you are conscientious about taking your supplements, you will ingest up to 30 mg of zinc per day—more than enough to boost your immunity. Check the nutrition facts on your preparations to calculate what you take.

Omega-6 Oils

Omega 6-oils deliver linolenic and gamalinolenic acid to the body that help to create the hormonelike prostaglandin E1 or PE1, an essential contributor to a healthy immune system. The omega-6 oils do not behave like prostaglandins E2 and E3, which some research claims to suppress our immunity. If you use corn, soy, and sunflower oils, you will receive plenty of omega-6.

Coenzyme Q10

You will remember that the antioxidant coenzyme Q10 plays a powerful role in the health of the heart. It also diminishes the production of lipofuscin, an unattractive yellow waste that deposits itself in your cells over time: The degree of lipofuscin in your cells indicates age. Further, new research shows that coenzyme Q10 helps regenerate the immune systems of older mice—therefore, it may well be helpful to older people as well. The commonly prescribed dosage of Q10 is 30 mg, but if you suffer an immune-system deficiency, or if you are ailing and must strengthen your defenses, feel free to increase your intake to 100 mg or more. There are no known side effects to an excess of this coenzyme.

Vaccinations

There is an old, tried, and tested method for developing immunity against particular diseases. It is called vaccination. In many countries, children receive a variety of vaccinations as a matter of course, for example against diphtheria, typhoid, tetanus, mumps, and measles. In eugeria, the most common vaccination is against influenza, since older people are more prone to complications of influenza that may lead to death. A yearly flu shot helps to protect us.

The influenza vaccine varies from year to year, depending on the strain of flu that predominates. Currently, vaccinations are injected, but oral or nasal spray vaccinations are expected to reach the market soon.

Vaccines are effective at a rate of around 75 percent. Therefore, if you are over seventy, you should insist on a flu shot at the onset of winter or at least by the end of October.

If you are likely to be exposed to either tetanus, polio, pneumonia, or hepatitis A or B, then other vaccinations are also necessary. At your next annual visit, why not discuss your options with your doctor.

STRESS AND IDLENESS

This section looks at how we are caught between pressure and idleness . . . or between stress and boredom. Our modern lives preclude physical effort, especially if we live in big cities. Typically, we rise in the morning as late as we can, gulp down our breakfast, rush to work through the traffic (yelling at other motorists), and attack our assignments at a ridiculous pace. Lunch may be a measly sandwich at our desk, and then we are racing against deadlines before we rush home to dinner, or some tiresome entertainment. Or we collapse in front of mind-numbing TV.

The French have a term for it: *metro-boulot-dodo*: Metro-work-sleep.

In our heavily scheduled lives, we have little time for physical exercise, save the occasional stroll or ballgame. Yet, there is no denying that regular exercise is essential to health. And signing up at a health club is not enough. You must find time to go.

The Bad News about Retirement

You may look forward to your retirement: "Whoopee," you say, "I hate my job. The customers are demanding, my boss never satisfied, my subordinates are constantly thinking of ways to trip me up! I cannot sleep at night, my heart beats too fast. . . . But when I retire, I'll take long walks in the country, visit museums, play golf every day, do odd jobs around the house. . . . My life will be wonderful!" Forgive me, but I must disillusion you. Unless you prepare for retirement, these romantic activities will still elude you. Unless you have habitually exercised throughout your working life, you are likely to quit after your first round of golf. Either you'll have trouble finding a partner, or the sheer effort will put you off.

And while you will relish your first trip to the museum, soon those museum visits will become even less regular. You will begin to feel empty and lazy: Your spouse or your friends will have to drag you out. In the end, it will be almost too much effort to walk your dog around the block.

What about the restaurants? The shows? The exotic trips? Well, if you're rich, they are always an option, but retirement also spells a diminished income and a strict budget.

Interesting Activity Keeps You Young

For all its stressful annoyances and shortcomings, your life preretirement is essentially active. When you retire, you may give in to a sedentary life and the associated risk of boredom and apathy— and these are stressors themselves. It's not activity, but too much responsibility that generates stress, especially when you fail to realize your objectives. Without goals, your mind and body deteriorate. This accelerates aging, and accelerated aging is a shortcut to death. As an older person, it is essential you discipline yourself to stay active: Find a project or interest that engages your passion. In fact, physical and mental activity contributes to physical and mental health throughout life. Never let your age deter you. Keep interested and busy: It will keep you alive. Write a book, collect Japanese prints, learn a new language, take up the piano, start a small business. If you can make a little extra money on your new hobby, so much the better. If you cannot come up with your own project, why not enroll in night school or adult school at your local college? In fact, I suggest you find two hobbies: one for indoors during foul weather and one for outdoors that requires physical exertion. Whichever way you look at it, interests energize you: Once you are energized, you may well rediscover your passion for golf. With your increased vitality, you will probably make new friends at the club—enough friends to play with every day of the week.

The Golden Rules for a Stress-Free Life

If you can strike a harmonious balance between intellectual and physical activity, you have laid the foundations for a stress-free life. Add to this a supportive home, a circle of friends, and a rewarding spiritual life, and you have all the ingredients for a joyful retirement—and healthy eugeria.

Stress is often described as *le mal du siècle*, the ailment of the century. In 1950, a Canadian physician and educator, Hans Selye, proposed that stress was the body's response to harmful external stimulants. Stress is a phenomenon of adaptation that puts the organism in a state of alarm and defense, arousing our attention, stimulating evaluation and judgment, and activating the capacity of decision. These are beneficial effects of stress, but it has its negative effects due to overreaction.

Overreaction to Stress

Often, our physical reaction to external stimulus may be more harmful as the "danger" before us. Some individuals cannot handle difficult situations (such as confrontation) and become nervous, irritable, and even aggressive in the face of minor psychological threat. In these cases, stress induces insomnia, depression, violence, isolation, and addiction: Alcohol and tobacco are classic panaceas for stress-related disorders.

Physical Effects of Stress

At a biological level, the hyperexcitability induced by stress is expressed in noticeable physical symptoms. Have you experienced any of these?

- heart palpitations and chest pain?
- difficulty in breathing, caused by constriction of the larynx or chest?
- numbness and tingling in the fingers and feet, as well as cramps in the calves and other parts of the body?
- sexual impotence?
- headaches, colitis, and constipation?

Common Stress Factors

Except for rare cases of catastrophe, such as earthquakes in California, watch for:

- overwork
- conflict at the office
- dismissal
- divorce

- chronic disharmony between you and your spouse
- family problems
- death
- conflicts with parents or children
- bankruptcy, debts, or even instant wealth

The Biology of Stress

From a biological perspective, stress begins in the brain and follows the hypothalamus that activates the pituitary gland that secretes a hormone that activates the adrenal glands, until adrenal hormones are excreted, mainly cortisol and adrenaline, which are responsible for the clinical aspects of stress. Research shows the responsibility of acute stress in heart attack. In fact, a recent study of 129 survivors of heart attack revealed that 51 percent of the survivors were exposed to some severe stress during the twenty-six hours before the attack.

Coping with Stress

At its most basic, the treatment of stress is preventive. An obvious choice is to remove yourself from the stressful situation. Simplify your life. Meditate. Take up an enjoyable sport. Eat healthy, whole foods. Take long walks on the beach. Quit cigarettes and excessive liquor. Schedule a few peaceful breaks during your busy day. Do isometric or stretching exercises every two or three hours. Get enough sleep

In more severe cases, you may try behavioral therapy or even psychotherapy. From relaxation techniques to conflict resolution—there are many nonpharmaceutical ways to address your tensions.

The cognitive approach adds a complementary dimension to relaxation: In fact, we quite often interpret situations as stressful where "reframing" might save us from internalizing catastrophic situations that in reality might not exist. Cognitive therapy helps patients be aware of these wrong interpretations due to overgeneralization or catastrophism, and guide them toward a better understanding of their own reactions in order to manage the triggers that lead to unwarranted stress.

Pharmaceutical Options

In the end, pharmaceutical treatments can also help: From vitamin B shots, sedatives, antianxiety medication to antidepressants, there are many options. If lifestyle changes fail to relieve you, then consult your doctor.

PART III
ATTAINING EUGERIA

CHAPTER EIGHT

Nutrition

BASIC DIET GUIDELINES

Four basic rules should govern your diet in eugeria:

1. Eat healthy and varied food.
2. Don't overeat.
3. Establish a healthy weight and maintain it.
4. Learn to read the nutrition facts on food packages.

Calorie Counting

Your ideal calorie intake is linked to your activity level, that is, how much energy you burn every day. Here are some guidelines that most accurately apply to those over age seventy.

Women: 1,600 to 2,000 calories per day
Men: 1,800 to 2,300 calories per day

Ideal Weight

As I already discussed in "weight excess" (see page 50), if you are only five to ten pounds overweight, it is more important in eugeria to maintain a steady weight than to traumatize your system

by struggling repeatedly to drop those excess pounds. The key is
to follow a sensible diet.

Proportions of Carbohydrates, Proteins, and Fats

I recommend the following proportions daily for older people:

Carbohydrates: 300 to 400 g
Proteins: 70 to 80 g
Fats: 45 to 50 g

Particular Dietary Needs

Basic guidelines aside, it is always important that we account for
particular needs and certain conditions. For example, high levels
of uremia, caused by excess protein, clearly indicate you should
cut your intake of protein. If you suffer from diabetes or insulin
resistance—sometimes the fault of inadequate chromium—you
must necessarily monitor your intake of carbohydrates. Similarly,
if high cholesterol is your particular problem, be sure to reduce
your consumption of fats.

Calculating Your Food's Components

How do you know if you are eating the correct proportions of various food groups and calories? You can consult the nutrition table in
the appendix, page 231, that breaks down the components of most
common foods. Otherwise, always read the nutrition facts on commercial food products that include the gram value of proteins, carbohydrates, fats—with cholesterol—minerals, and vitamins, natural
or added. Numbers and percentages are determined on a per-serv-
ing basis, so take note of the quantities a serving contains.

Watch Your Fat Intake

If you are in good health in eugeria and your cholesterol level is balanced within normal limits—up to 2.7 g per liter—you should still watch your fat intake and eat plenty of fresh fruit and vegetables. Fruit and vegetables contain polysaccharides that lower your insulin levels (see chapter six), besides all-important vitamins and digestive fibers.

Meat, poultry, fish, and cereal provide necessary proteins, but know that close to 20 percent of red meat is made up of fat. Choose low-fat milk products as a good source of protein and reduce your meat intake. Milk is also rich in calcium, which is essential for your aging bones.

FOOD DO'S

Unless you suffer a particular condition, and if your food choices are fresh and healthy, there is no need for a specialized diet in eugeria. However, I advise the following.

Snacks

Have two small snacks between your three main meals every day. You also need to replenish the liquid in your body. A large glass of water is best, otherwise try sugarless black or green tea.

Fruits and Vegetables

Eat five servings of fruits and vegetables every day. Fresh produce is best, but if this is impossible, choose frozen over canned foods.

Vegetables are often called *enzyme inductors* because they help to produce certain enzymes in our bodies. Fruit and vegetables also furnish the body with all-important vitamins and fibers. In fact, eat them raw when you can, as a number of vitamins are destroyed during cooking.

Cruciferous Vegetables

Broccoli, cabbage, cauliflower, brussels sprouts, watercress, radishes, and turnips contain chemicals called *phenols, indoles,* and *isothiocianates* that have life-saving properties: They help to protect us against colon and breast cancer.

Carrots and Spinach

Carrots and spinach are especially rich in carotenoids and protect against malignant tumors of the lung, the breast, the bladder, and the esophagus.

Garlic and Others

Include garlic, onions, shallots, chives, and asparagus in your meals as often as possible. Garlic, and to a lesser degree, this whole family of vegetables, contain a miraculous ingredient called *allicin.* The worst thing it does is give garlic its peculiar smell. The best thing it does is rev up our immunity. Allicin also reduces cholesterol, acts as an antibacterial, antiviral, and protects the brain from mental malfunction, such as memory loss and distorted thinking. Garlic's antioxidant properties are remarkable and are a key component in our fight against cancer. If you cannot stomach the taste or the smell of the great "stinking rose," then there is a simple solution: Take garlic in pill form.

Soy

Why do the Japanese live longer than other ethnic groups? By all accounts, it is their diet. The Japanese eat many soy products.

Current research proves that soybeans contain two potent antioxidants—genistein and daidzein—which help prevent cancer. In particular, these antioxidants lower the sex hormones, thereby reducing the incidence of breast and prostate cancer. Try defatted soy milk with your cereal, miso soup as an appetizer, and tofu with stir-fried fresh vegetables. The Japanese also eat seaweed and algae—both of which are rich in minerals, especially iodine.

Fats

A balanced intake of fats is best in eugeria: For those over age sixty, include the following proportions of fatty acids in your diet:

Total percentage of calories consumed as fat 30%
   Percentage of saturated fat   20
   Percentage of monounsaturated fat 60
   Percentage of polyunsaturated fat   20

The ideal salad dressing should be made with rapeseed oil, which contains 8 percent saturated fat, 62 percent monounsaturated fatty acids, and 30 percent polyunsaturated fatty acids. Olive oil is higher in monounsaturated fatty acids, but still makes a healthful and tasty condiment. Sunflower oil is richest in polyunsaturated fatty acids. However, there is current debate suggesting that polyunsaturated fatty acids produce the greatest percentage of unhealthy free radicals, despite the fact they are always accompanied with their own antidote—vitamin E. In the end, let your choice of oils depend on the kind of fat you consume in the rest of your diet, your cholesterol levels, your consumption of antioxidant-loaded foods, and your personal taste! Remember that heat alters the composition of most polyunsaturated oils. For this reason, choose oils high in monounsaturated fats for cooking (see chapter five). In fact, the healthiest way to prepare your food is to steam your fresh vegetables or brown them quickly in a skillet or wok with a dash of olive oil.

Fish

Eat fish at least four times per week, especially fish low in fat and calories, such as whitefish and snapper. However, don't deny yourself fatty fish, such as tuna, salmon, herring, and sardines, because these fish are rich in omega-3 oils. Remember, omega-3 oils are marvelous combatants against cancer and heart disease. Occasionally, try carefully selected, fresh raw fish if you can, since cooking destroys polyunsaturated fats. I suggest sashimi, tuna tartare, marinated salmon, and my personal favorite, marinated tuna prepared the Tahitian way.

High-Fiber Foods

Whole-wheat or whole-meal breads, cereals (especially bran), pasta, and beans are all excellent sources of the insoluble fibers that prevent constipation. More importantly, fiber helps prevent polyps, those precancerous tumors that develop on the intestinal wall, as well as colon and breast cancer.

Dairy Products

Include one dairy product with every meal. Try low-fat milk, cottage cheese, or yogurt—all of which are lower in fat than hard, yellow cheeses. Besides providing the necessary calcium, yogurt also provides digestive ferments—such as acidophilus—that contribute to the health of your intestinal flora. If you are inclined toward lacto intolerance, try goat-milk products. Goat cheeses and yogurt are more easily tolerated by many people. Butter and eggs are rich in minerals—especially calcium—and liposoluble vitamins such as E and A. Unfortunately, both are also high in calories and cholesterol, so limit your intake.

Organic Foods

Where possible, select organic meats, fruits, and vegetables. This way, you will avoid the dangerous nitrates and chemical additives which can cause cancer. However, make sure you wash your organic foods carefully. Occasionally, they carry dangerous bacteria and parasitic microorganisms, which can cause severe food poisoning and weaken your digestive system.

FOOD DON'TS

Processed Foods

Avoid industrially processed foods as much as possible. Most processed foods contain far too many nitrates and salt. As they originate from chemical fertilizers, nitrates are commonly transformed into nitrosamine, which is carcinogenic. Disturbingly, nitrates have penetrated the earth's water table and have begun to show up in our drinking water. As far as possible, insist on fresh or deep-frozen products and prepare them yourself.

Salt

Limit it: It makes for high blood pressure. Also, under experimentation, salt significantly reduced the life span of rats. Some scientists disagree with this ban on salt, so if you have no special problem, like hypertension or water retention, use salt to your taste.

Red Meat and Fat

Beware of red meat: It is overly rich in saturated fat. At least remove the skin of the chicken and any excess fat on your steak before cooking. If you cannot bring yourself to cook without fat, then peel away the skin and extra fat before eating.

Fried Foods

Never fry your food, especially in butter. Never order fried foods in restaurants. At best, sauté or grill your vegetables and fish in olive oil. Barbecued meat or foods cooked on a rotisserie can be carcinogenic. In fact, the burning grease that results from these cooking methods produces the same kind of tar found in cigarettes!

Avoid rich sauces and fancy "cuisine" loaded with fats and too many calories. Rather, select lightly cooked fresh products. Remember that excessive heat can destroy healthful vitamins, not to mention good flavor.

CHEW! ENJOY!

Finally, importantly, eat slowly! Take time out to enjoy a healthy meal in good company. Eating is a pleasure, not only a necessity. Food can ground you and calm you. Never underestimate the value of a fresh, wholesome meal as a way to buck stress.

ALCOHOLIC DRINKS

Drink red wine especially, but do not exceed the allowed dose. If excessive alcohol causes drunkenness, lesions of the heart muscle, and irregular heart rhythm, how can minor consumption protect us from heart attack? In an experiment in which participants consumed 39 g of alcohol daily, it was found that their concentration of good HDL cholesterol increased by as much as 17 percent.

What's more, the alcohol decreased their LDL levels, implying a decreased risk of heart attack by 40 percent!

Red wine is a lot more than water and alcohol! As red wine grapes soak in their own juices and then ferment, the juice—and future wine—is infused with health-saving tannins from the skins, pits, and stalks. Tannin contains components called *proanthocyanidols* which, surprisingly, are energetic free-radical scavengers. They belong to the family of flavonoids that combat cancer. They also act as antivirals and protect against radiation damage from the sun and X rays. As antivirals, they combine with viral proteins and neutralize them.

Do you need more? Have a small drink! For wines richest in tannins, enjoy Pinot Noir, Alicane-Bouschet, Cabernet Sauvignon, or a fine Merlot.

Some California researchers claim that red wine produced in the Napa Valley contains acetylsalicylic acid, that is aspirin, at high enough doses to prevent blood clotting.

Other Alcohol

Besides red wine, what alcohol should you drink? Whiskey dilates the arteries, and a few researchers insist that its tranquilizing action assists against stress! Certain American research studies that propagate a reasonable consumption of alcohol use whiskey in testing and recommend it for health, but at the level of no more than two drinks per day. For my part, I favor red wine, not least because I was born near Bordeaux! Moreover, the studies in support of red wine's antioxidant properties are numerous and extensive. It makes one wonder whether red wine is responsible for what is known as the "French Paradox." Despite incredibly fatty cuisine, such as foie gras and cassoulet, the French have far fewer heart attacks than do Americans obsessed with fat-free food!

How Much Wine?

As long as you don't have to work or drive in the afternoon, try a small glass of red wine at lunch (3.5 oz with 10-proof alcohol is the equivalent of 10 g alcohol.) Otherwise, opt for water, and drink no wine at all.

In the evening, before dinner, treat yourself to a light whiskey, say 1.5 oz, 12 g of alcohol. Otherwise, enjoy a glass of champagne or wine: Usually, this translates into 12 g of alcohol. With dinner, one large glass of red wine will give you 5 oz, or 18 g of alcohol. In short, I recommend a total of 30 to 40 g of alcohol per day— no more than half a bottle of wine. However, as you get older, you may find this may be too much, since alcohol affects us more as we age. Begin by omitting your drink before dinner. And women, reduce the recommended amount by a third anyway.

If you have never consumed alcohol, dare I suggest you bring it into your diet? If the idea is repugnant to you, or you are in- clined toward alcoholism, then your abstinence is for good rea- son, and I do not insist. Black and green teas are excellent substitutes for red wine, as both are full of antioxidant rich tannins. Even bet- ter, recent Japanese research shows that chocolate contains the same healthful flavonoids.

Alcoholism

The benefits of drinking small amounts of alcohol are clear and conclusive. However, this is no reason to drink without restraint. Alcoholism is a plague. It ruins your physical and mental health, not to mention your family and social relations. A good quality red wine is no longer medication if you do not limit the amount you take. During holidays and celebrations, do not overindulge. Occasional overdoses affect your heartbeat and your blood pressure, due to abnormal contraction and expansion of blood vessels. This stress on your body can lead to heart attack and stroke . . . a brutal interruption to a short-lived euphoria.

Water versus Alcohol

Finally, never drink alcohol to quench your thirst. Wine is a pleasure, a reward, or a medication, but it is no substitute for the liquid you need to replenish your body. Wine will never hydrate you. In fact, drink at least one and a half liters of water per day: That is almost ten glasses.

SIMONE

If we have no weight problem or disturbed metabolism of carbohydrates (diabetes), proteins (uremia), or fats (high cholesterol), do you seriously think, Dr. Lintilhac, you or I need to count our calories and weigh the food we eat? I concede I have seen you occasionally read the nutrition facts to check what you were eating, but no more.

On the other hand, someone who has a problem of obesity should be under the care of a nutritionist or a dietician and not embark by him- or herself on a fancy diet.

If you have diabetes, kidney problems, or high lipids, your doctor will prescribe a diet and eventually a medical treatment. If you are in good health and your weight is normal, I think you can eat whatever you like and satisfy your appetite. If you weigh yourself regularly and maintain a stable weight, it proves that the amount of food you ingest is adequate.

Of course, it's important to remember the recommended foods:

- *Skimmed milk, yogurt, and cereals*
- *Five servings of fruit and vegetables daily*

- Fish four times a week (especially fatty fish like salmon and tuna)
- Remember also that you should not eat too much fat, especially cooked or fried
- Outside of that, you should feel free to eat any kind of food you choose in reasonable quantities.

How do I manage my own cooking? Although I am French, don't expect me to give you any fancy recipes. After marrying Dr. Lintilhac, I was lucky to have a cook all my life, or at least a maid who could cook for me.

I am not a good cook and what is worse, I hate to cook, spending several hours preparing a meal that will be eaten in a few minutes.

I can sew, build, and decorate a house; paint; write; but don't ask me to cook.

Now that I live mostly in the United States, I have a maid who comes four days a week, but she does not cook; on the contrary, we have to cook lunch for her, and she has a good appetite.

Here are some of my little tricks to avoid having a lot of cooking to do while applying the rules of proper nutrition:

- I use, as much as possible, my steam cooker for vegetables; it is so easy, quick, and healthy.
- I buy two roasted chickens at the supermarket. We eat one with steamed vegetables the first day.The next day I prepare a chicken salad with the one that is left.

The salad is made of greens (sometimes endives), tomatoes, celery, onions, diced apples, and nuts. The sauce is made with olive oil, wine vinegar, and Dijon mustard. At least once or twice a week, we eat sushi of different kinds and seaweed salad that you find in all good supermarkets. At least once a week I prepare Tahitian style marinated fish, a delicious dish that conforms to the recommendations of modern dietetics.

Although I don't like to cook, I do like to set a nice table with my china, silverware, and crystal. I think even the most austere diet tastes better if it is served in a more festive manner. The meals should be eaten together by

Marinated Fish, Tahitian Style

red tuna, cut into cubes
1 quart water
2 tbsp salt
1 juice of one lime, per serving
1 onion, diced
1 carrot, diced
1 tomato, diced
1 cucumber, diced
salt
pepper
Coconut milk, olive oil, or lime juice
chopped green onions

Cut fresh red tuna into cubes. Pour one quart of water plus two tablespoons of salt into a salad bowl. Soak the tuna in the salty water for fifteen minutes. Using a sieve, discard the water.

Press the fish in a clean cloth to remove the excess liquid.

Squeeze the juice of one lime per serving over the fish and mix well until the liquid is evenly distributed. Marinate the fish for another five minutes. Afterward, pour off the excess lime juice. Finally, add the diced onions, carrots, tomato, and cucumber. Sprinkle with salt and pepper to taste. Mix well and let stand for a few minutes.

Before serving, add plenty of coconut milk, but be warned, coconut milk is high in saturated fat. Otherwise, try olive oil, vinegar, or extra lime juice.

Stir well; sprinkle with chopped green onions, serve, and enjoy.

the whole family and guests (if any). Take your time to chew and savor the dishes, and keep the conversation going. Conviviality is the best aid to a poor appetite or slow digestion. Since they are recommended by the faculty, I am very touchy on the choice of red wines. In the United States, we belong to a club that presents an excellent selection of California and French wines at reasonable prices; this greatly facilitates the choice of your everyday wine. And, in addition to being beneficial to your health, wine also boosts your morale. The Bible already stated: "Bonum vinum laetificat cor hominis." (Good wine makes the heart of man rejoice.) Red wine should be uncorked at least thirty minutes before the meal to let it breathe, and should be served in a decanter.

I read today in the L.A. Times that garlic, contrary to the common belief, does not reduce the level of cholesterol in the blood. This is the conclusion of an apparently serious study by German scientists. There is only one catch! The study is based on twenty-five cases, which eliminates any statistical significance. To illustrate this point, let me tell you a little story:

When my husband was preparing his book on cosmetic surgery, he wanted to know the percentage of the different operations he was performing, so he asked me to go through the last 100 operations he had done and note the percentage of each type. To our surprise, I came up with 0 percent breast operations, but we knew that he practiced these operations quite differently. So he asked me to look at the 1,000 last operations and the final percentage was 15 percent. Like we French like to say: There are three ways of lying: by intention, by omission, and by statistics. This is how, for example, statistics of breast cancer associated with hormone-replacement therapy show an incidence ranging from −20 to +40 percent. So, maybe after all, garlic does not lower blood cholesterol, but we need further studies based on much larger numbers of cases.

MULTIVITAMIN, MULTIMINERAL SUPPLEMENTS

We have already discussed how deficiency in vitamins and certain minerals can cause extreme health troubles. The official view claims that supplements are redundant, because we can get all the nutrition we need with our food. While this is true most of the time, I am amazed that this dogma would deny older people products that are at best life preserving and at worst only harmless. Some vitamins and trace elements are superior antioxidants. In fact, I propose we take more vitamins and trace elements than the FNB recommends. Remember that the Food and Nutrition Board is the government body that sets U.S. guidelines for daily dietary allowances. While I strongly support a cornucopia of dietary supplements, my intention in this chapter is not to address specific health problems or particular deficiencies. Here, my approach is preventive. If you include the supplements I recommend, your body will receive at least what it needs. Any additional vitamins and minerals that come in your food are no cause for concern. It is only important that you ingest enough to sustain a healthy eugeria. Often, a mineral or vitamin deficiency is not detected in its early stages, yet it still compromises the health of your body. A course of supplements ensures against and corrects such invisible problems.

Minimum versus Optimum Intake

Not only do vitamin and mineral supplements protect against cancer and disease, but with their eutrophic effects, they also contribute to our all-around well-being. The so-called "minimum" recommended daily allowance of vitamins and minerals we may receive from our diet is measured in terms of what we need to sustain life. Supplements give us an edge. First, they ensure we receive sufficient nutrition, and second, they bolster good health and extend life.

Calculating Dosage

Since we must consume at least twelve different vitamins and about as many minerals every day, we cannot get caught up in arbitrary doses. The most efficient way to ensure you receive adequate amounts of useful vitamins, minerals, and trace elements in balanced proportions is to consult the recommended daily values (RDA) set by the government bodies concerned. Or refer to the vitamin and mineral chapters in this book! With a little research, you will be able to find a single product—such as an excellent multivitamin and multimineral supplement—with the power to feed your entire body.

USP *Standard*

When choosing your supplement, look for brands that have been approved by the USP (United States Pharmacopoeia), which sets quality standards and tests market-bound supplements. Once in a while, make sure you change brands. This way, if your supplement lacks any essential component, the imbalance is corrected by your alternative product.

Understanding Measurements

Doses are measured in:

IU	International Units
mg	milligrams = 0.001 g
mcg	micrograms = 0.001 mg
% daily value:	percentage of the recommended daily or dietary allowance

In effect, your daily intake should amount to 100 percent of the RDA.

Vitamins A *and* D

Be careful not to overdose on vitamins A and D (see chapter six). If you take a multivitamin supplement as well as an antioxidant tablet, note that vitamin A will be included in both. Further, both vitamins A and D are often added to processed foods, such as milk products and cereals. During a period of several months, do not exceed a total of 10,000 IU of vitamin A and 800 IU of vitamin D.

Chromium and Zinc

Do not select any multivitamin, multimineral product that excludes zinc or chromium. However, do not exceed 30 mg of zinc every day. And check on the content of selenium in both your multivitamin, multimineral and antioxidant supplements. Your total selenium intake should not exceed 300 mcg.

In addition to your multivitamin and multimineral, take the following supplements regularly.

Calcium

Your optimum amount of calcium is rarely received per multivitamin, multimineral formulas. Therefore, take an additional calcium supplement of 1,000 mg, especially if you are a woman resistant to hormone replacement therapy. Calcium guards against osteoporosis.

Magnesium

Some people insist on magnesium supplements. The "miraculous" magnesium acts against heart disease, high blood pressure, weakening bones, and fights free radicals. However, multivitamin, multi-mineral supplements typically supply no more than 25 percent of our recommended daily allowance. You should take a supplement of 250 to 500 mg magnesium every day.

B *Vitamins*

Most multivitamin, multiminerals do not furnish enough all-important B vitamins, so I think it is useful to regularly add a B complex supplement to your vitamin intake. We can reduce homocysteine levels in our blood by taking vitamins B_6, B_9, and B_{12}. These Bs prevent artery clogging and heart attacks. They also work with the other B vitamins—especially B_1—to stimulate energy, reduce the physical effects of stress, fight fatigue, and promote mental clarity. As an alternative, while it is no longer fashionable, I recommend brewer's yeast as a source for all the B vitamins. Every other month, take a vitamin B complex daily and the next month, brewer's yeast (in capsules or powder form), which is rich in vitamin B, selenium, and chromium.

ANTIOXIDANTS

You will remember that antioxidants battle free radicals, which contribute to aging and all types of pathology (see Theories on Aging, page 10). Inflammation caused by bacteria, toxic chemical substances; radiation; viruses; and some common conditions, such as arthritis, all make free radicals. In turn, free radicals exacerbate cell inflammation.

Clogging of the arteries causes obstruction and blood clots. In turn, these blockages trigger infarction (blood diffuses in the tissues where the blood supply has been interrupted) and a flooding of free radicals to vessels in trouble. Moreover, a sudden rush of blood occurs when the blockage is released. This "reperfusion" produces more health-defying free radicals than the blockage itself.

There have been conclusive reports that free radicals actually attack our bodies genes, and therefore contribute to the onset of cancer. They are even responsible for cataracts. Here, their unchecked production is usually triggered by extreme sun exposure.

The Body's Defense Against Free Radicals

For all their health-defying negativity, free radicals actually happen normally and are useful in some physiological functions, such as the respiratory process and antibacterial defense. To an extent, so that they don't go beyond this role, our bodies develop their own defense against them. Our weapons are endogenous free-radical inhibitors, enzymes that we produce ourselves.

Superoxydedismutase (SOD)

Superoxide dismutase (SOD) is found in the body in two separate forms. One contains copper and zinc—which have their own antioxidant properties—and a lesser form works with manganese. In a little-known treatment of osteoarthritis, some doctors inject SOD directly into the joints of their patients. Also, since SOD quells the sudden onset of excessive free radicals, other doctors use SOD injections in aftercare treatment for heart-attack patients. SOD is not widely used yet, because it is mostly impractical. Though it can be bought as a food supplement over the counter, its value is questionable: Specifically, its action is very short–lived, that is twenty minutes at best, and its bulky molecule is unlikely to penetrate through the cell membrane.

Glutathione Peroxydase

Glutathione peroxydase, in conjunction with selenium, is also an excellent antioxidant. Glutamine itself an antioxidant, is a popular source of glutathione as it is easily absorbed by the body. Catalase is another good endogenous free-radical inhibitor. However, all these endogenous antioxidants are only effective when we ingest sufficient amounts of their cofactors. In other words, you need copper, zinc, manganese, and selenium for them to work. Fortunately, a good multivitamin, multimineral supplement—as well as extra selenium—is likely to offer high enough doses of these cofactors.

A free-radical scavenger is anything able to capture a damaging bachelor electron without being destroyed or transformed into a free radical itself. These are the "good guys"—and are characterized by their taste for free radicals. A few are particularly partial to specific free radicals

Exogenous Antioxidants

While some free-radical scavengers are produced in our bodies, we ingest exogenous free-radical inhibitors with certain foods. These are carotenoids—vitamin A; tocopherols—vitamin E and selenium—vitamin C and flavonoids.

Carotenoids
Vitamin A   Though beta-carotene is the most active carotenoid, other members of the carotenoid family are also good antioxidants. Tomatoes are rich in lycopene; corn contains zeaxanthine, and you'll ingest canthaxanthine when you eat broccoli or green cabbage. However, of all the carotenoids, beta-carotene most easily transforms into vitamin A when your body needs it. At the same

time, all carotenoids inactivate free radicals, particularly unpaired, single-oxygen atoms. For this reason alone, it is important to include carotenoids in your diet: Without a partner electron, oxygen atoms are both common and dangerous.

Tocopherols   The most active tocopherol is alpha tocopherol—commonly known as vitamin E. Vitamin E is fat soluble: It penetrates the double layers of the cell membrane and fortifies its defense against maverick free radicals. This gives vitamin E a peculiar antiaging characteristic. Also, when it is ingested along with selenium, vitamin E further increases our defense against cancer. Once vitamin E captures a destructive free radical, it mutates into a free radical itself, but in this form it becomes far less reactive. Subsequently, when the practically impotent free radical meets vitamin C, it is transformed once again into vitamin E.

Vitamin C   While vitamin C regenerates vitamin E, it has its own antioxidant properties. For one thing, it protects your skin from the damaging effects of the sun. However, in high concentrations, say in excess of 10 g, some studies claim that vitamin C actually engenders free radicals.

Flavonoids   Also described as proanthocyanidols or pycnogenols, these potent antioxidants are most often found in red wine, black and green tea, chocolate, citrus fruit, and pine bark.

Methionine and Cysteine

Methionine and cysteine are amino acids, combined with sulfur. They are lesser-known but effective antioxidants and are available in supplement form.

Coenzyme Q10

The chemical structure of coenzyme Q10 is similar to that of vitamin E. Specifically, it helps transform nutrients into energy inside our cells. That is why we find high concentrations of coenzyme Q10 in the heart muscle, because our heart needs high energy. A coenzyme Q10 deficiency often results in heart disease. Still, coenzyme Q10 also reinforces our immune defenses, and deficiency most often occurs when excess cholesterol is made. Cholesterol production inhibits its synthesis.

Glutathione

Glutathione is the active element of an enzyme called *glutathione peroxydase*. It neutralizes the free-radical hydrogen peroxide, which we recognize in hair dyes and as disinfectant in mouthwashes. Glutathione is regenerated by the enzyme glutathione reductase with vitamin B_3.

Why Do We Need Antioxidants?

There is no conclusive proof that antioxidants enhance all-around good health. However, their singular benefits are demonstrated in countless studies. What if we cannot prove that they prolong life? Since most progressive-minded doctors insist that antioxidants increase the quality of life, isn't quality of life the fundamental tenet of a vibrant eugeria? What is more important? Comfort and energy, or racking up years?

You will remember that I introduced you to 122-year-old Jeanne Calment in the beginning of this book. Although her mind seemed to be clear—she must have had good genes—she sat immobile and almost deaf and blind. In this condition, was her life worth preserving? I suggest antioxidants may have eased her long life. While normal, healthy nutrition can provide all our vitamins, let me remind you of our task in eugeria. More than supplying our bodies with sufficient reserves, we seek to defend ourselves against deficiencies caused by oxidative stress. With this goal in mind, our vitamin requirements exceed the limits that merely maintain us.

Research into antioxidant behavior is relatively new. A number of studies have not occurred under controlled conditions, nor have they included large enough cohort pools. Of the results published, some researchers hail antioxidant supplements as death-defying miracles, yet others suggest antioxidants are inclined to pose problems. The sensible approach is not to use antioxidant supplements as treatment for diseases or to take single antioxidants without the others. Taken in groups, each seems to support the others' efficacy.

In 1994, French scientists launched a study called *Suvimax—SUpplement VItamins, Minerals, and AntioXidants*—in which 15,000 out of 100,000 volunteers monitored the effects of a supplements program on their health for eight years. No results have been published as yet, but the medical profession is eagerly awaiting them.

I believe eight years are not long enough to judge results. Supplements are preventive elements, not medications. After all, cancer can take twenty years to develop; atherosclerosis begins early and takes some years to appear. It is unreasonable to expect useful conclusions until fifteen or twenty years down the line. Still, one thing seems clear. Antioxidants do no harm to us. And it is never too early to prepare for eugeria. To paraphrase the French philosopher Blaise Pascal, "When we bet on the existence of God, we have everything to win, and nothing to lose." It is the same for antioxidants.

Which Antioxidants? What Dosage?

Since most of the antioxidants are vitamins (E, C) or provitamins (A, beta-carotene), the amount of each you ingest in your food and multivitamin supplement is negligible compared to antioxidant supplements.

Be judicious. Measure the total amount you are consuming by checking the labels on all your supplements. You can receive optimum amounts of antioxidants in a single tablet, but if you want to make up your own menu, try the following per day:

Vitamin E	400 mg
Vitamin C	500 mg
Beta-carotene	20 mg
Pycnogenol or other flavonoids	50 mg
Selenium	100 mcg

Take 120 mg of methionine and 300 mg of cysteine daily from time to time. While I endorse many supplements, you do not need to take everything, always, and at the same time!

Also take:

Coenzyme Q10	30 mg (If you have a heart condition, many doctors suggest you take more.)
Glutathione	2 to 4 mg in powder form

Choosing a Supplement

These are the major antioxidants. Reasonably, you should not exceed 1 g (1,000 mg) vitamins E and C, though higher doses of vitamin C have been promoted and tolerated. And while excess vitamin A can be toxic, you are unlikely to overdose on beta-carotene. Also, do not exceed 300 mcg total dose of selenium, especially as you will ingest at least 70 mcg with your food anyway.

Zinc, copper, and manganese comes per your multivitamin, multimineral supplement. If you take antioxidants, never forget to take your multiminerals, since these elements act in synergy with antioxidant enzymes.

I recommend you select a formula that provides all the elements in one preparation. There are many antioxidant complexes available in the United States, and all in approximately the same composition. I take a single tablet that matches my own recommendations, but you may prefer a formula distributed between two separate tablets. Take one in the morning and one with your dinner.

Oxidative Stress

If you are in a state of "oxidative stress," whereby you suffer inflammation, high cholesterol, or you smoke, drink, and are exposed to air pollution, increase your dosage of vitamins C and E. Remember vitamin C regenerates vitamin E. In addition to the dosages I outline above, take:

Vitamin E   400 mg
Vitamin C   500 mg

Take additional supplements later on in the day, say when you eat dinner. Since excess vitamin C is excreted rapidly, splitting your doses helps maintain constant levels of C in your blood.

SIMONE

I am not here to discuss the doctor's orders. I don't have the scientific knowledge to make my own decisions, so I take regularly each morning:

multivitamin, multimineral supplement
antioxidants formula with extra C (500 mg), extra E (400 mg)
calcium-magnesium
B-complex or brewer's yeast
salmon oil or lecithin

gingko biloba or ginseng
eventually coenzyme Q10, *or* DHEA

I *take all of them with my breakfast in the morning, which makes it easier
since I don't have to bother about taking supplements for the rest of the day. I
don't have a problem digesting these supplements, but I have a plea to the
manufacturers of these food supplements: Please don't make tablets so bulky
and hard to swallow. Don't try to put all the ingredients of your antioxidants,
multivitamins, multiminerals, or calcium-magnesium into just one tablet,
especially one with square angles. Several times I almost choked on one such
tablet that was blocked in my throat. I have tried to help them go down, eating at the same time some yogurt or a bite of banana, with some success.*

Why *don't you make two tablets for the same dose and give them the
shape of a football, which would make them much easier and less risky to
swallow. It would also allow your customers to take them at different times
of the day, if they prefer, thus prolonging their action.*

*Quite often I suggested to my husband that he give the names of the
brands he recommends with their composition. But he answered that it
would be unethical and would sound too commercial.*

ESSENTIAL AMINO-ACID AND
ESSENTIAL FATTY-ACID SUPPLEMENTS

Strictly speaking, these are not vitamins, but just the same, these
essential amino acids and fatty acids must be supplied in certain
quantities and proportions by food to the organism that is unable to synthesize them.

Essential Amino-Acid Supplements

You can find protein preparations, in drugstores or health stores,
whose labels give their composition, and for the most serious, the
"aminogram," which will allow you to make your choice by check-

ing that they contain the essential amino acids in the desired proportions (see Essential Amino Acids, page 57). In the older person in eugeria with normal nutrition and weight, such supplementation is of no use.

On the contrary, it is necessary in the aged in a state of denutrition, be it as a result of insufficient intake, unbalanced nutrition (depression, bereavement, medication) or a defect of absorption.

It can be useful in the older subject who has a fat excess and a muscle loss to help him or her lose weight and to build up muscle mass.

Essential Fatty-Acid Supplements

If you follow the recommended diet by eating fatty fishes (rich in omega-3 fatty acid), preferably raw, or if you eat salads prepared with rapeseed and soy oil (omega-3), or corn and sunflower oil (omega-6), it is not necessary to take any supplement. If not, you can find capsules of onagre oil (evening primrose oil) or fish oil to add to your food. Fish oils are especially indicated in cases of abnormal elevation of the triglycerides in the blood.

PREVENTION (AND TREATMENT) OF MENTAL AGING

Aging of the brain, if it implies deficits other that a certain slowdown of thought and benign memory loss, should be an obsession for anyone reaching the age of eugeria. All physical handicaps of age are negligible compared to the mental deterioration striking some older persons. But this deterioration is not inevitable; Dr. J. L. Robine, a French physician who has studied more than 25 percent of living French centenarians, came up with a theory: "The brain ages much more slowly than the body," he said. "Further, in the absence of illness, I suspect that the brain does not age at all." This goes against the traditional paradigm of aging but lends encouragement to the concept of eugeria.

Conventional wisdom proposes that an aging brain brings mental decline and loss of memory. Certainly, our thinking slows down, and we experience normal, tolerable, and benign loss of memory as we grow older. However, when mental deterioration accelerates rapidly, this is a crisis for us in eugeria.

Brain aging actually begins in our youth. From childhood, 100,000 neurons—brain cells—die every day and are never replaced. Brain cells do not multiply! We compensate for the deficit with what doctors call "cerebral plasticity." Our receptors and synapses—the connections between our brain-cells—actually multiply. And this multiplication keeps our brain going. Dopamine is a neurotransmitter, a chemical substance that help transport messages between our brain-cell synapses and also from brain cells to other organs. Between the age of twenty and seventy, our dopamine levels decrease by as much as 40 percent. Many scientists contend that the problem of communication between our brain cells is the most significant contributor to rapid aging. This idea has some merit, but we should never ignore the health of the blood supply to our brain or any changes in its metabolism. Be sure to engage in preventive measures, and always be watchful. Many diseases trigger intellectual and memory deficits such as Alzheimer's disease or vascular dementia.

Prevention of Mental Aging

Just as we exercise our bodies, we must exercise our minds to keep our brains fit. Memory and reasoning exercises keep our synapses functioning and can activate new ones. First, eliminate controllable toxins from your diet, such as tobacco and excess alcohol. Be cautious with sleeping tablets and antianxiety treatments. Not only are these preparations addictive, but they suppress brain activity. You have every good reason to quit them progressively, but consult your doctor before you do.

Sleep Disorders

You will notice that sleep disorders, such as insomnia, increase with age. Before you resort to medication, first try a few nontoxic methods. Reduce your consumption of coffee and black tea, especially in the evening. Exercise more during the day, and wind down at night with relaxing hot baths, guided relaxation therapy, meditation, or yoga. If you must medicate, try melatonin instead of barbiturates or other hypnotics. And remember, depression is a major contributor to disturbed sleep patterns, so ask your doctor if you need counseling before you resort to aging hypnotics.

Supplements

Vitamin and mineral supplements boost brain activity, and antioxidants protect the brain cells from free radicals.

B Vitamins

The B vitamins, especially vitamins B_6, B_9, and B_{12} reduce high levels of homocysteine. While homocysteine contributes to atherosclerosis, it also negatively affects the cells of the brain. Choose a supplement with magnesium, which functions in synergy with the B vitamins. Also, alternate you supplement with brewer's yeast every second month.

Soy Lecithin

Phospholipids are an important component of brain tissue, and since lecithin and soy oils are rich in phospholipids, you can supplement your diet with soy-based lecithin to support your brain-power. Look for a brand rich in the especially potent phospha-tidylcholine.

Ginseng

Some traditional Chinese herbal therapies straddle the line be-tween drugs and food supplements: The ginseng root contains compounds called ginsenosides, valuable minerals, and vitamins B and E. Though it continues to be seen with skepticism in the West, ginseng has been used in China for thousands of years. It improves resistance to fatigue, strengthens the immune system, and stimulates intellectual activity and memory. Mostly, you can find it in health-food outlets, in capsules of fine powder. Take at least 500 mg and no more than 1 g daily. Excess ginseng—say 2 g daily—can cause nervousness, insomnia, skin rashes, diarrhea, and even temporary hypertension. Extreme excess—up to 10 g— triggers inflammation of the brain arteries. Irrefutably, then, gin-seng affects them!

Ginkgo Biloba

The magnificent ginkgo biloba tree is indigenous to China, but today it is grown all over the world. The leaves contain compounds called *flavone glycosides* and *rutin* which support the blood supply to our tissues and protect cell metabolism, especially in the brain, ears, and eyes. Ginkgo biloba also contains antioxidants, which, specifically, tackle free radicals in our brain cells. Traditionally, the herb is prescribed for intellectual and memory loss in older peo-ple, ear problems causing deafness and dizziness, retina disease causing blindness, as well as poor circulation in the lower limbs.

Ginkgo biloba is available in tablet form or solution. In eugeria, I recommend you take 120 mg per day. Only abstain if you experience side effects such as headache, rashes, or digestive disorders.

Without side effects, these traditional Chinese herbs strengthen your hand against cerebral aging. Since there is no need to take both simultaneously, I propose you alternate between the two remedies. Take ginseng for a month and ginkgo the next two. In the end, ginkgo biloba appears to be the superior supplement. Most people prefer it.

Omega-3 Oils

Raw fish, oily fish, and plant-based omega-3 oils are all important to the health of the brain. However, unless you are a strict vegetarian or have digestive disorders, I doubt you need supplements of essential fatty acids. However, if you do choose to supplement, take flaxseed or fish oil. I recommend salmon oil: 1,000 mg soft gels, two daily.

Treating Cerebral Aging

Are you forgetful? Do you have trouble concentrating? Do you suffer shakiness, abnormal muscle jerkiness, dizziness, or insomnia? Are your symptoms getting worse? My best advice here is to see your doctor, who will select from four classes of drugs. Interestingly, the drugs that treat brain aging are most often distilled from the active components of a wide range of herbs.

Cerebral Vasodilators
Cerebral vasodilators dilate the blood vessels of the brain. Many cerebral vasodilators are derived from rye ergot. The most common is hydergine. Others, such as naftidrofuryl, are synthetic com-

pounds. Procaine, once used as a local anesthetic, is best known nowadays under its brand name Gerovital, originally formulated by a Romanian, Dr. Anna Aslan. Her formula, also a synthetic compound, became famous in Europe as a rejuvenator. Later, another brain-activating drug was derived from procaine—diethyl amino ethanol, best known as Deanol.

Other drugs act on the *metabolism of the nerve cells*. Vincamin is derived from the periwinkle. Piracetam is a synthetic compound improving the metabolism of brain cells.

Psychotonics enhance the brain's activity. Others act on the neurotransmitters and are defined as *cholinergic* or *dopaminergic*.

If, after investigation, your doctor detects the onset of a neurological or mental disease such as Alzheimer's, Parkinson's, or any other brain-vessel damage, he or she will treat you accordingly. Rest assured that a great number of old people never suffer pathological memory or attention loss. Still, there is no reason to wait for severe symptoms before you initiate prevention or treatment. Indeed, many "brain" drugs can be used for prevention! Discuss your options with your doctor or gerontologist, who would be most knowledgeable as it concerns your individual case.

CHAPTER NINE

General Hygiene and Sex in Old Age

EXERCISE

Current studies show that exercise decreases your risk of heart attack by 50 percent. Consider one particular study that shows Americans would save themselves $3.4 billion in yearly medical costs if they all only walked three to five miles a day. This study even accounted for the cost of increased physical strains, such as sprained ankles! Yet another study specifies that walking three miles per day reduces your risk of heart attack by 64 percent, and those who exercise regularly are 50 percent more likely to survive between ages sixty-five and eighty-four, than those who do none. Exercise improves the quality and length of your life. It is also cost effective! Before embarking on an exercise program, schedule a checkup with your cardiologist. Many older people have at least minor degrees of coronary obstruction. Also, if you take beta-blockers for high blood pressure, then your pulse may be slower. Once you establish your heart is in good health, then enjoy your favorite sports well into eugeria. Unless your doctor preaches otherwise—because of the reasons given—try to increase your heart rate by 50 percent during aerobic activity.

Aerobic Exercise

Isotonic, aerobic exercise increases oxygen consumption and strengthens your heart. Try walking, swimming, or bicycling. A stationary bike or treadmill protects you from the elements and accidents. Jogging is good for well-trained enthusiasts. If you have never jogged, it may not be advisable to begin now. I still remember seeing on French TV, President Carter trying to run a semi-marathon. The cameraman caught him out of breath, completely exhausted, right at the moment he was abandoning the effort. And the panting, staggering American leader was thus broadcast for the whole world to see, making me wonder if he had taken a bigger personal risk on this day than he did during his whole presidency facing terrorist attacks. If you have never jogged, it may not be advisable to begin in eugeria.

Overexertion before you are physically ready is dangerous. Beside the strain on your heart, research shows it unleashes many free radicals.

Walking

My favorite form of exercise is walking, especially after age seventy. Set off at a sustained pace, but try to avoid walking in traffic—exhaust fumes are toxic. During his first term, President Clinton once jogged through the streets of Paris. The stunt was good for publicity, but for his health, he would have been better off jogging in the Bois de Boulogne. There he could have exercised in a place full of greenery. Bois de Boulogne is away from the traffic, yet it is still in the city. Walk three to five miles a day or swim for thirty to forty-five minutes. If you enjoy golf, refuse the cart ride. Rather, walk briskly between every hole.

Weight Training

For increased muscular strength—not to mention good looks—begin a program of weight training. But remember that weight training is not as essential as aerobic activity. An exercise trainer can help you establish a healthful routine. One point to keep in mind, however: In eugeria, the weights should not be so heavy that you experience sudden surges in blood pressure. At this point in life, your heart cannot take it.

Tai Chi

Finally, begin every day with limbering exercises, such as tai chi, chi qong, or yoga. Tai chi and chi qong are ancient Chinese disciplines and yoga hails from India. Basically, tai chi focuses on mobility and balance, yoga on flexibility, and chi qong on energy. None of these exercises needs a special place or equipment to practice—you can easily do them all in your living room. Undoubtedly, they keep your joints and muscles well oiled. Also importantly they strengthen your breathing.

Breathing

The first and fundamental tenet of flexibility training is to inhale and exhale in deep, abdominal sweeps. Though we habitually breathe in short, unconscious puffs that do not fill our lungs, deep breathing fully engages our consciousness. This is highly beneficial for us in eugeria. As we age, our rib cage loses elasticity, and our capacity to take in enough air is compromised. See that you receive enough oxygen by conscious breathing—to the point where you feel the air pressing down on your abdomen.

Stretching

Simply moving your joints can combat the stiffness that comes with old age. Slow, harmonious movements that focus on balance—which is often disturbed in older people—along with focused breathing, slows you down to focus on the moment at hand.

As you put your other problems aside, you will find that these exercise, relax, and destress you.

First learn these disciplines from a master, either in class or from a video, then you can continue your program at home. In the end, you may find your classes are most enjoyable. For one thing, they are social. For another, your teacher will help you get the best from your workout.

SIMONE

When I was young, I practiced dance and gymnastics. Later, from thirty to fifty, I was a fervent practitioner of yoga. I liked to swim long distances in the sea during our summer vacations. I seized any opportunity to walk in Paris, shopping or going from one place to the other. It is always a pleasure to walk in Paris, admiring the monuments or looking in the windows of the luxury shops. When I arrived in Tahiti at fifty-five, I decided to do some more active training. Aerobic exercise was then highly fashionable, so I joined an aerobic class with much younger people, and I could follow the rhythm pretty well, but this was too much for my aging knees. I had to undergo the removal of the meniscus of my left knee under endoscopy. I recovered full mobility in a few months, but I abandoned aerobics, which quite obviously was not suitable for my age. I went back to my walking habits, never taking my car to go places in Papeete, in spite of the poorly maintained sidewalks. I also swam two or three times a week in our pool.

At over seventy, coming to Los Angeles, I developed a technique: Everything I do, I consider a form of exercise. For example, whenever I dress, I try to work on my balance by standing for awhile on one leg. When I have to reach for something on a higher shelf, this becomes a stretching exercise. If I have to tie my shoes, I don't bend my knees, I just bend forward, and so on. Every time I have some housework to do, rather than a chore, I consider it like exercise (and it is exercise!). I like to garden, and it too becomes quite a workout. I admit that this is all a point of view, but it changes the way you consider things and also the way you practice them. In short, act young. Walk briskly instead of dragging your feet. We have a gym in the building, and though its good exercise, I never go on the treadmill or a bicycle, which I consider boring, even with the TV on.

I much prefer to walk with my husband along the quiet streets around our home, enjoying the nice houses with their lawns and flowers and the blooming jacarandas along the sidewalks. My husband likes to use the well-heated swimming pool every day, but I must confess that I use it less frequently. I avoid the sun, and besides, my makeup and hair do not like the water.

ACTIVATE YOUR BRAIN!

Exercising your body keeps your mind fit! Still, though improved circulation promotes improved mental clarity, it is not enough to keep you mentally healthy.

Keep Abreast of the News

Retirement often condemns older people to mental and physical inactivity, but it is essential to keep your mind engaged. Your first defense is not to lose contact with the outside world, even if you find the news irrelevant or somewhat depressing. Read the newspaper, watch educational programs on TV, write letters to friends. Crossword puzzles and brainteasers are excellent methods for keeping your memory and powers of reasoning in shape.

Work on a Computer

Computers have games, word processing, accounting, and organizing programs—all wonderful tools to keep your mind busy. Never assume that you are too old for it. Computers are not so complicated that you will never learn. Ask your children and grandchildren to give you a hand! The possibilities inherent in computers are endless: You can manage your money, compose poems, maintain an inventory of your record collection—the choices are almost unlimited.

Enjoy Your Odd Jobs

Never pass up the chance to tackle odd jobs. Don't throw out and replace that broken toaster—fix it! Install new bookshelves. Take up cooking or a craft. I know a number of men who are artists of tapestry! If you appreciate art, take a watercolor class, join a poetry circle, why not try an unusual musical instrument? If learning new skills does not interest you, then take the time to listen to beautiful music of your own taste.

Unplug Your TV!

Whatever you do, don't aimlessly sit and stare at TV. On the occasion you do, choose a thought-provoking movie, an educational documentary, or a worthy news program. And only turn on the tube during the time of your broadcast.

Family

Your relationship with your family is important. If you are married and are still with your spouse, then you are lucky. If you receive regular visits from children and grandchildren, you are doubly blessed. As you get older, you might find them intrusive, but do not complain. Not only is solitude an anathema to a happy eugeria, but kids make you young! Don't hesitate to play with your grandchildren. Talk to them. What does it matter if they humiliate you now and again!

Friends

If you have no family, your friends can provide you with as much support. As you get older, your circle will shrink. It is difficult losing lifelong loved ones, and I do not expect you to try to replace them. However, new acquaintances are better than no friends. Therefore, go out of your way to meet new people. Enroll in a bridge club. Join an organization for senior citizens. Introduce yourself to other members of your golf or tai chi club. Volunteer for a charity that inspires you. Take a few university courses . . . the possibilities for meeting new people are endless. You could even take an organized tour or set off on a cruise.

If money is a problem, simply go to a dance. Not only are dances excellent exercise, but they are great ways to meet spirited people. What's more, they are fun and occasionally offer opportunities for romance. A number of dances are organized by senior citizens, and I know a few couples past seventy-five who fell in love at one of these events.

Which brings me to the next section on sex in eugeria.

SEX AND OLD AGE

As long as your sex life is emotionally gratifying, regular sex is a boon to your health. Indeed, your sex life can be a means to gauge your physical, hormonal, and mental well-being. Having said that, an active sex life is no precondition for good health and longevity. If you are celibate, there is no need to worry that you have a health problem.

Men

After sixty, you need more time to reach an erection, which is less firm than when you were younger. Moreover, you need more time to reach orgasm, which is often shorter. Typically, older men lose their erections more rapidly, take longer to be aroused once again, and, unlike young studs, once old men reach orgasm, they rarely have another round in the gun. Don't worry about this! Ask any woman—quality lovemaking succeeds over quantity!

Impotence

You can experience impotence for many reasons, just as unsatisfactory performance and disappointing experience is not uncommon with advancing age. At least 20 percent of sexual dysfunction in men over sixty is attributable to reduced production of the male hormone testosterone. In other cases, atherosclerosis restricts the blood supply to the genitals and inhibits one's capacity to sustain an erection. Similarly, various medications prescribed in eugeria produce the same problem. These include beta-blockers for hypertension, neuroleptics for depression, and hypnotics prescribed for sleep disorders. Fear of failure actually exacerbates sexual dysfunction. Fortunately, psychotherapy and sexual counseling can help put you back on track. For the less severe impotency, testosterone treatments can help immensely. If you must take medication for more serious health problems, then the perfect solution is less easily reached. You can change medications or stop them altogether, although you should exercise this alternative only under advisement. Your last resort? Simply resign yourself to a less active sex life.

Treatment Options   Besides testosterone injections, another solution comes also by injection. You can inject the deep erectile tissues of the penis with a special solution of papaverin or prostaglandin E_1. This option is appealing, but beware: Some men suffer painful and prolonged erections long after they want it. Also, with constant use, scar tissue nodules often develop on the shaft of the penis. If you are afraid of the injection as an alternative, try introducing a kind of small suppository (muse) into your urethra.

Another method uses a specialized vacuum pump to draw blood into the erectile tissue. Once your penis is filled, tie a tourniquet to the base of the shaft to keep it erect. Sadly, this approach is not always effective. For one thing, you risk sustaining only partial erection and failed ejaculation occurs as much as 40 percent of the time. Also, this method has a disquieting side effect, that is, a cold penis. Some loving partners have been known to complain!

Unless you are highly motivated—say your partner is much younger than you are, or your sex drive is high—there is a good chance you will give up on these procedures in time. For this reason, the new pill Viagra has become an immediate success.

First tested for angina, the drug failed to solve heart problems but turned out to bolster flagging male potency. Fortunately, Viagra became recently available, having obtained the green light from the FDA for the treatment of male impotence. It is delivered only with a doctor's prescription, which is a good thing, since there are a few contraindications (especially vasodilators used for the treatment of angina), and some cases of death have been reported after its use. If you need it, ask your doctor before using this new miracle drug.

Permanent Solution   A permanent solution may be the use of reinforced or inflatable silicone implants. The procedure works like this: A bendable metal rod included in a silicone implant is inserted into the shaft of the penis. The downside to this surgery is that you must live with a permanent erection. However, for discretion and comfort's sake, you can always bend your penis to one side. Otherwise, tubular, inflatable silicone implants come with a small pump of saline solution. You can pump saline solution into the inflatable implant at will. Then, when sex is over, the saline solution drains back to the pump. Silicone implants seem to work fairly well. They are permanent, ready to use, and, for the most part, men find them satisfactory.

Women

Except for women treated with hormones, vaginal secretion decreases significantly with the onset of menopause. Where sex is concerned, vaginal dryness can make intercourse painful and ultimately inhibit the ability to experience orgasm.

Lubricating jelly is your first solution. Otherwise, begin treatment with estrogen, topical or taken internally, as early as possible after you begin menopause. An absent libido or lack of a partner are most older women's only sexual deterrents. There is little to stop women from having sex in old age.

Singles and Couples

Couples who enjoy an active sex life throughout their lives usually prolong their interest well into eugeria. On the other hand, if you have been celibate for many years, it may be difficult to be sexual again. Still, even when men experience impotence, there is no reason to give up on sexual activity. After all, penetration is not a prerequisite of a good time! Further, masturbation is always an option. In keeping with the opinion of Jocelyn Elder, our beleaguered ex-Surgeon General, I believe sex for one is both safe and pleasant! I am sorry this wisdom cost Elders her job.

Research reveals that older people rediscover masturbation without any prompting by government bodies. Sex therapists Christensen and Gagnon claim that older women practice solo sex readily, regularly, and without shame. After all, isn't it better than lusting after young innocents or entering dangerous encounters that could lead to diseases like AIDS?

Interestingly enough, I recently read a news story: "Man, ninety-five years old, tests sero positive after encounter with prostitute." While I was—of course—sad to read of his dilemma, I was also secretly pleased a ninety-five-year-old libido was on public record.

Then I read on: Oh no! "The prostitute bit the man's hand to force him to let go of his clutch on his wallet. That is how she infected him."

What is closer to the truth is that as age progresses, libido decreases. Perhaps we should be pleased. No longer are we a slave to our sex drive. No longer are we driven wild by temptation. Now we can settle into well-earned serenity. And when our obsession with flesh has abated, what do we have left? As Elvis says, "Love me tender, love me true!" What could be more wonderful than that?

PHYSIOTHERAPY AND SPAS

In Europe, people patronize spas as a matter of course. The composition of the local mineral water makes these getaways great centers of healing and rejuvenation. Every spa has a particular specialty: While some revitalize your general well-being, others treat high blood pressure, rheumatoid arthritis, skin disorders, or asthma, depending on the singular mineral content of the area's water. There is no spa that I know of that concerns itself exclusively with issues of aging. However, many common health problems are also the problems of progressed age. For example, in France, Brides les Bains is built at a particular altitude in order to treat rheumatism and obesity, both of which are concerns in eugeria. Another, known as Royat, deals with circulatory problems, especially in the brain and retina, and their treatment approach is thought to aid against cerebral aging.

Thalassotherapy

Some spas specialize in thalassotherapy—cure by seawater and algae—which is extremely rejuvenating. Thalassotherapy spas are located on seacoasts in areas especially rich in minerals (iodine in particular) and algae. Water used in the therapy is unpolluted because it is pumped from deep within the sea, then heated and poured into Jacuzzis and pools, where, under the supervision of physicians, therapists massage you and guide you through invigorating exercise and mobilization programs. However, there is no need to go to a spa to gain the benefits of mineral-rich seawater. A regular swim in the ocean is far less expensive and a wonderful form of aerobic exercise.

In fact, proximity to the sea is good for eugeria. As the waves break onto the beach, they negatively ionize the surrounding air. An ion is an atom that has a charge, and the effect of ionization is a strong charge of energy. Before a thunderstorm, your heavy, restless or depressed feelings are due to the positive ions in the air. Negative ions are more abundant at high altitudes and at sea level, but not in between. Take three weeks in the mountains or by the seaside and you will be energized. Or, if you can afford it, take a trip to a spa. If you cannot, perhaps you can locate a whirlpool nearby. Throw some algae powder into the rollicking water, sit back, and enjoy. You may even buy a simple appliance that emits negative ions, and ask a loved one to massage you while you breathe in the healthy, negatively charged air. Spas are developing and becoming more popular in the United States. I hope this book will encourage them.

CHAPTER TEN

Treatments for Eugeria

Beyond diet, hygiene, vitamins, and antioxidant supplements, you can try pharmacological antiaging approaches. However, these must be prescribed by your doctor alone.

The best way to weigh a new drug's efficacy is to consider its corresponding potential for harm. Doctors perpetually weigh advantages against drawbacks when they administer medicinal products.

Following hundreds of thousands of test cases, two particular treatments are currently popular. One of these is hormono-therapy for postmenopausal women. The other one is aspirin. Both decrease mortality caused by cardiovascular ailments and certain cancers. They also, importantly, improve the quality of life in old age.

In the following pages, we will also look at some less confirmed hormone treatments including:

- Testosterone prescribed for older men
- Growth hormone
- DHEA
- Melatonin

Though all are heavily promoted as miracle cures, not enough time has passed, nor has enough research been conducted, for us to be sure of their efficacy. At this point, we only have a few hundred studies to draw on.

HORMONE REPLACEMENT THERAPY
FOR MENOPAUSE

The level of female hormones drops considerably after menopause, and replacement therapy consists of giving feminine hormones (synthetic or natural), by injection, orally, or through the skin. Hormone replacement therapy is probably one of the most controversial therapies of our era. So I will be up front about my position. I support it. If you are an older woman, consider hormone replacement therapy as a boon to your health . . . as long as you remain free of contraindications.

Menopause is a momentous stage in a woman's life. As it signifies the end of her reproductive period, it comes with enormous hormonal upheaval. Menopause is the gateway to a woman's old age. It brings with it discomfort: Hot flashes—especially at night—fatigue, mood swings, and vaginal dryness. Miraculously, these symptoms disappear after just a few days of hormonotherapy.

Osteoporosis

In advanced years, women lose bone density, which often results in osteoporosis. This unhappy condition usually begins seven to eight years after menopause and affects 30 percent of untreated women. It begins with depleted calcium reserves. Then, the resulting bone loss causes impaction of the vertebrae and loss of height. Sufferers constantly risk fracture of their thigh bones and spine. Have your bone density measured when you begin menopause to calculate your propensity for this disease. While hormone replacement therapy is an excellent antidote for the symptoms of menopause, at least begin treatment by early postmenopause to suspend the onset of osteoporosis. Studies reveal that those who sustain hormonotherapy for ten years only lose bone mass almost ten years later. Indeed, there is no limit to how long you can continue treatment. Hormonotherapy is active for as long as you do it.

Atherosclerosis

In the childbearing years, women suffer significantly fewer heart attacks than their male counterparts. However, some studies show that women are more vulnerable to atherosclerosis and heart disease when they stop menstruating, and the statistics for heart attack between men and women become almost equitable. In effect, your female hormones protect you from heart disease. Though the length of menopause varies, the symptoms of menopause generally bother you during this time only. However, a significant number of women suffer hot flashes and depression well into post-menopause. Certainly, all women experience prolonged loss of moisture, especially in the vagina and skin. While these symptoms are irritating, they are far from health hazards. At worst, they affect the enjoyment of your eugeria.

To Have or Not to Have
Hormone Replacement Therapy

In a study of 8,881 patients, Dr. B. E. Henderson gave 5,000 women hormone replacement therapy. After ten years, he discovered those subscribing to treatment lowered their death rate by 20 percent over the women taking no hormones at all. Further, after fifteen years of therapy, the death rate decreased by 10 percent more. If you begin menopause before age forty-five, you are more likely to benefit from hormonotherapy than those who start later. In fact, your death risk decreases by 30 percent. Conversely, if you

begin menopause after age fifty-five, replacement therapy is probably wasting your time. Not that you are likely to die any earlier.
Quite simply, your body has no use for the extra hormones.

Henderson's Research Results

Of the pathologies that were positively influenced by hormone
replacement, Henderson's research tells us that women taking estrogen for four to fourteen years reduce their risk of death by heart
attack by 40 percent. They reduce their risk of death by stroke by
26 percent

They reduce their risk of death by various cancers: Specifically,
70 percent lower risk of death by cancer of the digestive tract; 15
percent lower risk of death by lung cancer; and 19 percent by breast
cancer. On the other hand, women increase their risk of dying
by cancer of the endometrium, that is, the inner membrane of the
uterus by three times if they take estrogen without progesterone.
Another researcher, Dr. Voigt, found that if women take progesterone at least ten days per month, they cancel their risk of cancer of the uterus engendered by estrogen therapy. In the United
States, most women take Premarin, composed of estrogen without progesterone. In France, doctors prescribe estrogen every day
and progesterone for ten days a month.

Risk of Breast Cancer

Hormone replacement therapy versus breast cancer is one of the
most controversial health topics today. First, Dr. Henderson found
that hormone replacement therapy reduced your risk of death by
breast cancer by 19 percent! Two French doctors, Dupont and
Page, carefully analyzed thirty-five other studies and came up with

less reassuring results. They took an average of all the reasonable research and found that your risk of breast cancer actually increases by just less than 10 percent. Similarly, from 1978 to 1992, the Nurses' Health Study looked at the risk of breast cancer and concluded that the risk was significantly increased when you take estrogen. And it is even greater when you take progesterone too.

Need I tell you the research is confusing? A more recent study, published in the *Journal of the American Medical Association (JAMA)*, concludes that women who take estrogen are not likely to contract breast cancer at all!

The Bottom Line About Hormonotherapy

Without question, hormonotherapy enhances the quality of your life and prevents osteoporosis and cardiovascular accidents. In fact, it lengthens your life to the tune of 20 to 30 percent. To vilify this treatment simply because it may contribute to the onset of certain cancers is unreasonable.

We must look for contraindications to the hormone therapy: Breast cancer in the family, no children, or late pregnancy. Since we can now detect genes that cause breast cancer, when in doubt it would be wise to look for these special genes in the genome.

Then if minor risks exist, conscientious monitoring leads to early detection and thus early treatment and probable cure. Still, as a woman, the choice is in your hands. Discuss your options and risk with your gynecologist.

Ask your doctor about the different types of estrogen and progesterone and length of therapy. It can take years, and can be permanent. Your personal schedule of checkups should include: Examination of the genitals and breasts by your gynecologist; regular pap smears and mammograms; and regulation of your cholesterol levels and fat consumption.

The Importance of Checkups

If you take hormone replacement therapy, schedule a minimum of twice-yearly checkups. Increasing your checkups is nothing more than a positive adjunct to treatment. Under conscientious monitoring, your doctor is more likely to detect irregularities and what may have caused them, after all, hormonotherapy is not the only possible trigger for cancer and disease. Your only concern is that you find and fight illness as soon as you can. If, God forbid, you do contract cancer, you will never be sure what brought it on. Certainly, hormonotherapy could be a factor, so could heredity, diet, and exposure to radiation, including radiation you receive with your mammograms. In France, only 12 percent, and in the United States, 15 to 20 percent of women currently use hormone replacement therapy. While many are ignorant of its benefits, others reject it because it is not natural. Yet others are put off by the hysterical fear of cancer surrounding it.

ASPIRIN

The German company, Bayer, first marketed acetylsalicylic acid—aspirin—as early as 1899 and controlled its distribution until World War I. Two decades ago, the drug had one purpose: to treat pain and fever brought on by common ailments—headache, influenza, rheumatism, and muscle strain.

Aspirin and Platelet Aggregation

Then, in the early 1970s, a plethora of studies signaled a breakthrough: Aspirin prevents platelet aggregation, that is, it stops blood clotting. Significantly then, aspirin helps prevent heart attack, stroke, and pulmonary embolism from blood clots originating in the deep veins. Historically, your problems occur when blood clots move from large arteries to smaller ones, where they become trapped.

The Physician's Health Study

The continuing Physician's Health Study observed 22,071 healthy doctors taking either 325 mg of aspirin or a placebo every other day for sixty months. Results showed a 44 percent decreased risk of heart attack in the group taking aspirin, compared to the doctors given a placebo. Significantly, the decrease only affected participants over fifty years old. Also, the doctors' risk of stroke increased very slightly. Actually, the researchers concluded that this increased risk was minor enough to render it insignificant. The message is simple: Whether you have already had an attack, or you have no previous history of heart disease, begin taking aspirin when you reach fifty. Not only does aspirin prevent heart attacks, but it is also important to secondary prevention (i.e., after you have already had a heart attack). It prevents stroke caused by blood clots. And though you slightly increase your risk of brain hemorrhage, your decreased risk of stroke more than outweighs your chance of that occuring.

Aspirin As an Anti-inflammatory

Aspirin is a nonsteroid anti-inflammatory that has none of the side effects associated with cortisone. Among other things, it works on sore and injured muscles, joints, tendons, headaches, toothaches, and earache. It is an excellent painkiller. Haven't you taken it sometime in your life? Significantly, even small doses treat the rheumatic pain that often ails older people. Also, many sufferers of arthritis attest to its soothing effect on sore joints and to a better quality of life when they take small doses of aspirin.

Aspirin and Colon Cancer

A major American study compared the incidence of death caused by colon cancer in subjects taking aspirin at least sixteen days per month to participants who took no aspirin at all. The conclusion? Of those taking aspirin, mortality by colon cancer dropped by 40 percent in men and by 42 percent in women.

Conversely, other studies report some bleeding in the lower bowels as well as the growth of scar tissue, which narrows the colon. Still, most research insists that aspirin helps prevent colon cancer. Not enough can be said for this simple drug. Without question, in enhances the quality of life for those in eugeria.

Contraindications

However, as any active drug, aspirin has a few side effects and contraindications: Over the years, doctors have reported incidences of gastric ulcer, a tendency toward hemorrhage in various diseases, and stomach lesions caused by its acidic nature.

For this particular problem, we have a solution: Try "buffered" aspirin, containing a neutralizing agent and coated aspirin that dissolves slowly and later in digestion. Occasionally, aspirin causes bleeding in the nose, gums, digestive, and urinary tracts. In the end, if you have any of the symptoms described, then simply discontinue your aspirin use.

Dosage

If you use aspirin as an anti-inflammatory, take it in high doses for short periods only, say up to 5 g for ten days. In the long term, particularly during eugeria, never take more than 325 mg. A minimum amount of 160 mg contributes to almost 90 percent inhibition of the enzyme TXA_2 that causes blood clotting; 300 mg stops TXA$_2$ 95 percent. For best effect, take aspirin continuously, but stop treatment at least a week before surgery. Blood that refuses to clot during surgery can be very dangerous.

In any event, neither begin nor stop a course of aspirin without first discussing treatment with your doctor.

TESTOSTERONE FOR ANDROPAUSE

The Male Menopause

While there are many studies devoted to menopause, doctors and researchers have only recently turned their attention to andropause. Male hormone levels decrease more slowly and are less physically detectable than they are in women. Not surprisingly, the subject of andropause is not only new, but extremely controversial.

Testosterone Replacement Therapy

Though the benefits are less spectacular than they are in women, some doctors advocate hormone replacement treatment for men. Where women receive estrogen, men take testosterone. However, more doctors support female hormonotherapy and few are convinced that testosterone replacement is as innocuous.

Prostate cancer is quite clearly linked to too much testosterone. This is a pity, because testosterone also contributes to increased muscle strength. That is why some athletes rely on male hormones as supplements. Testosterone helps men sustain sexual energy and prevents memory loss. When rats are administered with a single shot, they are noticeably better equipped to negotiate a maze than are rats who are given no shot at all.

If, as a man, you suffer any bothersome sexual dysfunction, you may consider testosterone replacement. As long as your prostate is in sound health, then testosterone supplementation is an excellent adjunct to a healthy eugeria.

GROWTH HORMONE

Growth hormone is secreted by the pituitary gland and its secretion decreases as we grow older. More than any other function, growth hormone assists in building our bodies, in terms of our muscles, tissues, and bones. Understandably, children produce more of this hormone than adults. However, be wary of popular stories praising growth hormone.

Research remains in its early stages, so it is too early to gauge long-term effects.

Growth hormone plays a key role in metabolism as it decreases fat tissue and increases the production of proteins and collagen. This function is important to us in eugeria, because it helps us lose fat and supports muscle growth. Also, growth hormone helps us retain certain minerals, particularly calcium, magnesium, potassium, and sodium.

Warning!

Remember how AIDS first appeared in blood products? In 1958, an American doctor, S. M. Raben, first advocated extracting natural growth hormones from human cadavers to treat hypophyseal dwarfism, a condition caused by deficient growth hormone. Tragically, the glands removed from the dead bodies were processed in pools of thousands, and batch after batch were contaminated with a deadly virus. Finally, in 1985, doctors identified a rare encephalopathy in dwarfs and slow-growing children who were given growth hormone. This was Kreuzfeldt-Jacob's disease, a tragic condition reminiscent of "mad cow" disease afflicting England in the late 1990s.

After the natural growth hormone was quickly withdrawn, it was replaced with a synthetic product from genetic engineering. Today, this synthetic growth hormone is costly and not yet available for antiaging. Further, fledgling studies are yet to establish cancer risks and other contraindications regarding this hormone.

Arginin

In the meantime, try arginin. Available over the counter, this potent amino acid actually stimulates your own production of the growth hormone.

If you are over sixty, take 8 g arginin daily for one month, then rest for six months. There is no reason to take it for extended periods of time.

DHEA: THE Treatment for Eugeria?

In January 1995, the French media was awash with stories heralding DHEA, Professor Emile-Etienne Baulieu's fantastic antiaging discovery. You will remember that the same Professor Baulieu invented RU 486, the controversial abortion pill. What is DHEA? Is it simple molecule that can keep us young and in good health until our last moment? Is this a miraculous shortcut to our goal of eugeria? Let me enlighten you.

DiHydroEpiAndrosterone—DHEA—secreted by our adrenal glands, is the precursor of male testosterone and female estrogen hormones. It is found only in humans and other primates. It circulates in our blood in the form of a sulfate, and its level in our blood varies as we age. It first appears at age seven, increases until we reach twenty-five, then it decreases. By age seventy, we are left with 10 percent of the DHEA we had in our twenties.

Low DHEA levels herald vulnerability to cancer and heart disease. When rats were given DHEA sulfate, they lost excess weight and almost lost their propensity for atherosclerosis and cancer. However, remember that rats do not live as long as humans, nor do they produce DHEA naturally. No question that we need comprehensive studies of the hormone on humans, and it will be years before we know all that we need to, including clinical precautions regarding DHEA's use.

Still, a colleague of Professor Baulieu's, Dr. Samuel Yen of the University of California, claims that older volunteers taking daily doses of DHEA enjoy increased energy, are more resistant to stress, sleep better, suffer less physical pain, and enjoy increased mobility in all their joints. More recent experiments suggest that DHEA supports the immune system and enhances the effectiveness of endogenous growth hormone, promoting healthy bone density and improved muscle strength.

Ironically, despite Professor Baulieu's fame, DHEA is not yet authorized for distribution in France, although it is sold commercially in the United States.

Certain DHEA supplements are sold in 500 mg tablets, but 500 mg may be excessive: In experiments, rats developed liver lesions when they were administered too much for their body weight. If you choose DHEA, stick to 50 mg daily. And make sure you are buying from a reputable source: Under analysis in some over-the-counter-products Professor Baulieu found no DHEA at all.

MELATONIN

The Other Miracle Drug?

Melatonin is secreted by the pineal gland, a pea-sized hormone-producing endocrine gland, attached to the underside of our brain center. We mostly produce melatonin at night. And, in the morning, when light hits the retina, the pineal gland ceases melatonin production. When production occurs, it flows to all parts of our body, especially the other endocrine glands. Depending on age, our level of nocturnal melatonin varies considerably. Maximum production occurs by age six and decreases considerably as we hit puberty. At age forty-five, it stabilizes at half a child's level and is halved once again by the time we reach eighty. Actually, a similar rate of reduction occurs with DHEA. However, unlike DHEA, melatonin is found in all living organisms. Melatonin regulates our harmonious rhythm with day and night and regulates sleep. It also regulates reproductive cycles in animals and their urge to migrate.

Melatonin in the Laboratory

Recently, researchers found melatonin had exciting antiaging effects. First, it is a potent antioxidant. In fact, it is one of few antioxidants able to penetrate protective spinal fluid in the brain cavity. As such, it protects mice against cataracts and some genes against cancer. When scientists cross-grafted the pineal glands of old and young mice, they found that melatonin boosts the thymus gland and even strengthens the immunity of older mice. Other experiments show that high levels of melatonin extend the lives of mice by almost three times. This particular study is significant. If the researchers' claims are confirmed, melatonin will be seen as a phenomenal medical breakthrough. It will take its place among very few substances that actually increase our maximum life span. At this point, melatonin is best known for helping us sleep! If you suffer insomnia or are subject to sleep disturbances, for example, night shifts or travel-inducing jet lag, melatonin can help. Take 3 mg at bedtime and if you cross time zones, take a second 3 mg if you wake up at night.

Side Effects

Aside from a few complaints about nightmares, we know of no undesirable side effects in regards to this hormone. A group of volunteers took high doses of 5 g per day for a full month, and the worst they suffered was minor stomach pain and loss of sleep! Ultimately, for its antioxidant and immune-boosting action, not to mention its possible effect on longevity, melatonin is a first-rate choice for eugeria. Having said that, the effects and consequences of long-term treatment remain to be seen, since we don't have the benefit of long-term research.

Dosage

Begin with one-half tablet of 2.5 mg for one or two months. Also, select a product that dissolves under your tongue. Sublingual absorption bypasses an initial passage through the liver, where the hormone is metabolized and partly destroyed.

If melatonin fails to help you, at least it won't hurt you . . . or your purse. A mere $4 will buy you a month's worth of 1.25 mg per day.

OTHER TREATMENTS

You may ask me, "How can you write a book on rejuvenation without discussing herbal treatments like royal jelly, aloe, algae, spirulina, cat's claw, etc.? What about all those miracle products I have heard about? Why don't you promote them?"

Here's my response: Eugeria has less to do with sensational cures or unreal means to rejuvenation. I am more interested in down-to-earth, well-used, and mostly proven and practical ways to aging in health.

Natural Foods Versus Processed Treatments

What's more, choosing sides between natural and industrially prepared products is completely unreasonable: Both synthetic and natural products are normally processed and the end result is the same. In other words, vitamin C is ascorbic acid whether you ingest it by orange juice or as a tablet. Do not assume natural foodstuffs are always superior to manufactured products. In some cases, nature can be dangerous. In fact, I prefer simple chemical elements obtained by extraction or careful synthesis, because this way a treatment's action is clearly defined, and dosage is easily and accurately measured. Even where natural products come to us in capsules or tablets, the strength of each dosage necessarily varies: The chemical content of plants always vary, depending on the soil in which they are grown. Even the soil in one place varies tremendously according to seasons and other conditions. Having said that, never underestimate the life-giving power of natural vegetable and animal products. The last thing you should do is skimp on fresh fruits and vegetables. Though we do not fully understand how the active ingredients in vegetables work, no one disputes their enormous health benefits. I am no enemy of natural products. I do not vilify nor forbid your use of pollen, propolis, royal jelly, algae powder, soy germs, etc. While these treatments are an anathema to most conventional medics, I do not doubt that many of them work. Still, eugeria draws on treatments that have been scientifically and methodically tested. Anyway, doctors habitually dispute one another's research, and opposing opinions abound whenever new treatments enter the market. You must simply make a choice. Look to those enjoying good health. This book reflects mine.

Remember Cell Therapy?

Many people ask me: "What about those celebrities, like the former Pope who received Niehans cell therapy from the Swiss professor? How is their eugeria? What has happened to cell therapy now?" If you remember, Niehans injected a suspension of the ground organs of immature sheep embryos into humans. In cell therapy, the embryonic organs used depended on one's ailment, for example arthritis, and other chronic degenerative diseases. However, some cell therapy simply rejuvenates, and shots included thymus, pituitary, and different endocrine glands, such as thyroid and sex glands.

Injected into the buttocks, the living cells migrate to and graft themselves to the corresponding human organ and revive it. Apparently, no serious scientific studies were ever conducted in the name of this method, neither by Niehans's supporters or his detractors—of whom there were many. Still, numerous patients reported increased energy and improved well-being, as well as healing of various ailments. However, cell therapy slumped when Niehans died and his organization reoriented itself toward beauty products.

Probably, the difficulty of managing embryo production, the risk of disseminating viral diseases, and the loss of its visionary caused the demise of Niehans's program. It went the same way as placenta implants, the brainchild of a Russian, Dr. Filatov. Like everything else, fashion plays a role in medicine too! Otherwise, why would certain medications, both efficient and well tolerated disappear and be replaced by cures that are no more effective? Remember that medicine production is very big business.

And to remain profitable, drug companies must continually entice us with newer, costlier products.

A SHORT GUIDE TO SUPPLEMENTS FOR EUGERIA

Multivitamin, multimineral
Take it every day without fail, especially if you are ill. Be sure it contains most of the vitamins and minerals at the RDA level. Check on vitamin D, zinc, and chromium. Change the brand every month or so.

Calcium 500 mg—magnesium 250 mg
Take 1 or 2 tablets every day in addition to your multi.

Vitamin B complex 100
Take every day for one month. Alternate with:

Brewer's yeast
Take every day, or continue B complex.

Antioxidants
Take every morning without fail especially if you are ill:

Beta-carotene	20 mg
Vitamin E	400 mg
Vitamin C	500 mg
Flavonoid	30 mg
Selenium	100 mcg

Or take an appropriately similar formula containing the same ingredients in one or two tablets.

In case of oxidative stress, smoking, drinking, high cholesterol, pollution later in the day, take one more:

Vitamin E 400 mg and vitamin C 500 mg

Add occasionally for one month:

Methionine	120 mg and cysteine 300 mg
Coenzyme Q10	30 to 50 mg
Melatonin	1 or 1.5 mg (sublingual)
DHEA	50 mg

Against brain aging, alternate insisting on Ginkgo:

Ginseng	500 mg or
Ginkgo biloba	60 to 120 mg

Take also
Lecithin (rich in
  phosphatidylcholine) up to 2,400 mg
Salmon oil   150 to 300 mg

Take the medication prescribed by your doctor.
For eugeria   aspirin, hormones

A TYPICAL DAY IN EUGERIA
FOR A RETIRED PERSON

7:00 AM: *Get up!* It is no use lazing about in bed. Spend thirty to forty-five minutes on tai chi, yoga, or other exercise of your choosing.

Shower Preferably with a firm scrub such as a loofah, exfoliating gloves, or a cloth. This helps circulation and rids your body of dead, scaly skin. Carefully brush your teeth, paying attention to massaging your gums. Apply moisturizing lotion to your face and to your body if your skin is dry.

8:30: *Breakfast* Prepare a meal of coffee or green tea. Avoid sugar or artificial sweeteners.

One fruit or unsweetened fruit juice

Cereal—preferably high fiber, such as bran, with skimmed milk or low-fat yogurt

Slice of whole wheat bread, toasted if desired, with butter (if your cholesterol is normal), fruit-sweetened jelly, or honey.

Take your multivitamin, multimineral, your antioxidants, and any doctor-prescribed treatments that must be taken at breakfast.

9:00: *Read the newspapers* Keep abreast of current events, the stock market, perhaps try the crossword.

10.00: *Get out of the house!* Take an hour's walk, swim, play golf, or go shopping.

11:30– *Relax* Back home, treat yourself to a small snack,
Noon such as a full glass of water or low-fat milk with carrots or celery. Kick back. Read or watch television, prepare the mid-day meal, and set the table.

12:30: *Lunch* Prepare a meal of:

Salad

Fish—grilled, steamed, or raw—or poultry, grilled without skin

Steamed vegetables
Low-fat cheese or yogurt
One fruit
One small glass of wine
Coffee or tea

1:30 P.M: *Read or watch TV*   This is a good opportunity for a "siesta." Always opt to rest after a meal, rather than exercise, as the process of digesting food causes hypotension.

2:30:   *Personal*   Housework, errands, chores, and odd jobs. Writing, studying, work on the computer, or creative endeavors such as music or painting.

4.45:   *Break*   Prepare a snack. Try a full glass of water, a cup of cold or hot tea, one fruit, a cup of low-fat yogurt, or a slice of whole wheat toast.

5:00:   *Personal*   Time for a family gathering or other social activity. Try charity work, chess, or card games, dress up to go dancing! Otherwise, choose a cultural activity, such as a visit to a museum or an educational lecture.

7:00 :   *Break*   One light whiskey or a glass of wine with nuts. Prepare the evening meal.

7:30 :   *Dinner*
Soup or hors d'oeuvres
Meat, fish, or pasta (only eat eggs if your cholesterol is normal)
Steamed vegetables or salad
Light dessert or fruit
Glass of red wine

Take the balance of your treatments for eugeria not taken throughout the day, as well as the balance of medications prescribed by your doctor.

8:30: *Entertain yourself* Watch the news or a movie, read or play cards. Go out! How about dinner, the theater, a movie, a concert, or a dance?

10:30: *Prepare for bed* Brush teeth carefully, clean face, and apply skin care treatment. Take melatonin if necessary.

11:00: *Good night!*

Part IV

Looking Young

CHAPTER ELEVEN

The Skin and Its Annexes

THE IMPORTANCE OF APPEARANCE

I have been a plastic surgeon for almost fifty years. Therefore, I am the last person to ignore issues of appearance, especially in eugeria. Looking young is important for our relationship to ourselves and to others. Not only is it satisfying to encounter a face in the mirror that is youthful and vibrant, but our appearance influences others, perception of us, and thus the way we are treated.

If we look young, we feel young. Good grooming has two benefits. Not only does it enhance our appearance but also our self-esteem. And, in itself, strong self-esteem is invigorating.

Many aging people complain that the deterioration of their physical image betrays their perception of themselves or their lifestyle. This chapter addresses this frustrating discrepancy.

Keep a Young Bearing and Good Deportment

A man walks down the street, and just before him walks an elegant young woman. Though he is a candidate for eugeria—or precisely because he is—his eyes follow the woman with interest. Suddenly she stops, gazes into a shop window, and he looks closer. Surprise! She is a lot closer to his age than he thought! The man has been "deceived" by her youthful bearing. A young bearing is a way to hold yourself and to move that reflects self-awareness more than chronological age. If you are a candidate for eugeria, you have every chance to maintain a young bearing, as long as you sustain a youthful spirit.

When you first meet a person, you notice his or her shape and weight. Then your eyes fall to the skin, especially to his or her uncovered face. After deportment, skin is the most important element in sustaining a healthy and youthful appearance. Skin is more than an elastic, pliable, envelope that separates our body from its environment. It has multiple functions.

First, it protects the body against invasion from water, bacteria, abrasions, shocks, and chemical agents. Second, it regulates temperature. It fights heat by sweating, and it fights cold with hair and fat stored in its deep layers. We actually breathe through our skin. It is an auxiliary organ of respiration as it is an auxiliary organ of excretion. We rid ourselves of toxins by perspiration. It stores reserves of fat. It produces vitamin D since the sun reacts with cholesterol stored in its layers. It absorbs alcoholic solutions and fats. That is why our skin is often used to introduce drugs to the body when we want to *bypass liver metabolism. Taken internally, drugs can sometimes be metabolized and changed to the point that their efficacy is adversely affected.

SKIN AGING

The Epidermis

The most superficial layer of skin is the epidermis. This includes what we call the *stratum corneum*, a film of dead cells with a horny consistency. As the stratum corneum flakes off through the years, it is renewed ever more slowly. Consequently, our epidermis becomes ever more fragile, more dry, and more rough. The other layers undergo less obvious changes: The cells of the basal, bottom layer reproduce more slowly. With age, the number of pigment-producing melanocytes in the basal layer decrease. Most noticeably, our hair gradually changes to gray, then becomes white.

Contrary to the thinning and atrophy of the skin that occurs during aging, consistent sun damage causes our outer layer to thicken and even proliferate in exposed areas.

The Dermis

As we age, the dermis becomes thinner and the number of elastic fibers that hold our skin together decreases. Collagen, the protein that settles between the skin cells and gives the skin its resilience becomes depleted. In fact, the collagen fibers thicken and fray like the fibers in fabric. Our skin loses elasticity. Blood supply to the dermis is decreased, our capillaries weaken, and we bruise more easily.

The Hypodermis

The subcutaneous tissue, or hypodermis, located directly below the dermis, is infiltrated with fat. With age, this fat is depleted in certain areas, particularly in the face and the back of our hands. At the same time, it becomes thicker in other areas, such as under the chin and on our stomach and thighs.

AGE-RELATED SKIN LESIONS

With age, skin becomes looser in both sexes, but if you are a woman, it will sag more because your skin is thinner. Certain lesions are particularly frequent in older people. Seborrheic keratosis, otherwise known as *senile keratosis* or "cemetery flowers" are brown wartlike lesions that appear most often on the back of your hands and on your face. Red and blotchy small tumors, otherwise known as *spider noevus*, are created by damaged blood vessels and appear anywhere on your body. Red, infected acnelike bumps that appear on your cheeks, chin, and nose are commonly known as *rosacea acne*. In older men, rosacea occasionally evolves into the spectacular *rhinophyma*, characterized by a thick and deformed lower part of the nose. Otherwise, age-related dry skin and seborrheic dermatitis characterized by irrepressible itching is highly frustrating because it is often resistant to treatment. And if you have spent too much time in the sun throughout your life, you run the risk of *actinic keratosis*—red and scaly bumps on the skin. Not only can these tiny bumps turn dark and unsightly, but they can penetrate into the dermis and trigger skin cancer. Therefore, if you have them, ask a skin specialist to remove them immediately. The sun is dangerous. Not only does it cause topical lesions, but its ultraviolet rays sap your immune system. In fact, your T-cell count drops after a day in the sun. Have you ever had cold sores after too much exposure? There is concrete proof of a weakened immunity.

Darkly pigmented moles, medically known as *pigmented naevus*, are vulnerable to melanocarcinoma, a skin cancer due to sun exposure. This form of skin cancer is not easily healed. It metastasizes rapidly and can even cause death. For this reason alone, keep close watch on your moles, and report any changes to your dermatologist.

CHAPTER TWELVE

Keeping Your Face Young

Want to age gracefully? Of course! Unfortunately, age rarely enhances our physical beauty. Jowls, turkey gobblers, bags under the eyes, deep wrinkles—these trappings of age invariably compromise our natural good looks. Further, recent scientific studies show that people who retain their looks are more optimistic, more social, have happier dispositions, and feel healthier than those who let themselves go. Moreover, others judge our age based on our appearance and make assumptions about us accordingly. Wouldn't you like the world to treat you as if you were ten years younger than you actually are? Wouldn't you hate to be treated as older? No doubt our morale and relationships are best served by looking as pleasant as possible throughout eugeria.

THE FACE

It all begins with your face. Every part of your face ages—your skin, the subcutaneous fat tissue, the fibrous tissues and tendons, your muscles, and facial bones. Apart from intrinsic aging, facial skin is exposed to external assaults, not to mention the wear and tear brought about by gravity and facial movements. Of all the elements that make up your face, your skin deteriorates first.

Sun Exposure

The most dangerous rays are the ultraviolet B rays. While ultraviolet A rays are less dangerous, they still harm your skin. It can even be damaged by excessive light and infrared rays. Wind, cold, dry air, and pollution are aging. Just look at the faces of long-term sun-worshipers, sailors, sportsmen, and workers who stay outside without hats: While their skin may be beautifully tanned, notice that it is thick, rough, and reveals cross-hatched wrinkles. Eventually, brown spots and deep furrows will underline their whole face, especially around their noses and eyes.

Cigarette Smoke

Cigarette smoke contains free radicals, which attack facial skin. Particularly, it affects the upper lip, especially in women, who have less hair than men. What's more, if you smoke, the normal vertical lines that come with aging will be accentuated by your repeated sucking on cigarettes.

Fight Wrinkles

If you are naturally very expressive and use your facial muscles to accentuate your feelings, or if you are victim to facial tics or bad habits such as frowning, squinting, or pulling down the corners of your lips, then no doubt your wrinkles will reflect your behavior. To save yourself from wrinkles, you can only use willpower and break the habit.

If you have been persuaded to exercise your facial muscles to prevent sagging, you should know that these exercises are not good for your skin. Repeated flexing of the skin actually causes the wrinkles you wish to avoid. Rather, try isometric contractions, or exercise your facial muscles with electric stimulation without

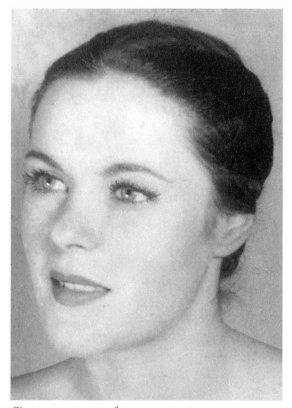

Simone at age twenty-five

deforming your features. In the end, gravity is one of your greatest enemies. Whatever stance you take—sitting, standing, even sleeping in any position other than on your back, gravity drags on your skin and makes it sag.

If you are a yo-yo dieter, that is, you habitually gain weight, then lose weight, then gain it again; your skin will ultimately show the effects of your dieting. Quite simply, your skin distends when you are heavier, then attempts to bounce back when you slim down. However, when you age, your skin loses elasticity and that is how you end up with sags on your face: It loses its capacity to spring back into place.

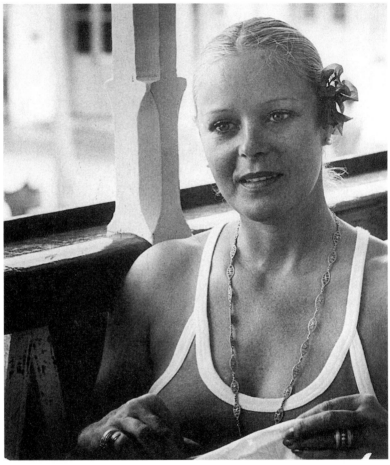

Simone at age fifty

Antidotes to Face Aging

First, maintaining your health and good estrogen levels is essential to preserving your skin. Second, be conscientious about sound skin hygiene. Only use nonirritating fat soaps to keep your face clean. Avoid cleansers that contain harsh chemicals, are too acid, or strip your skin of moisture. Cleanse with a dermatological abra-

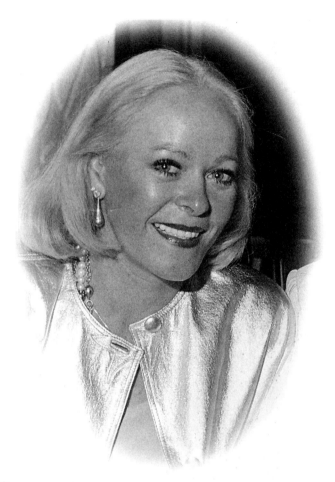

Simone at age sixty-two

sive cleanser occasionally, as this helps slough off dead skin cells that cause irritation.

Third, protect your face from the sun. Your natural pigmentation determines how much sun your face can tolerate. No matter how dark you are, never sun yourself at midday, when the ultraviolet B rays are strongest. Also remember: Though water and snow may be cooling, neither protect you from burning. In fact, the sun reflected off snow and water makes it extra potent.

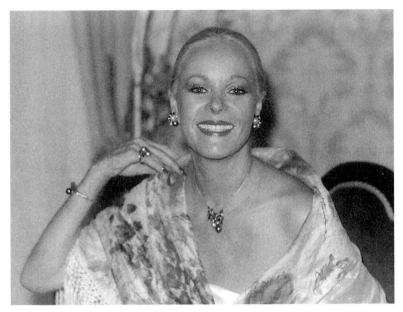

Simone at age ~~seventy-three~~ oixly five

Sunscreens

Your best defense is always to wear a sunscreen on exposed skin, particularly on your face. Apply total blockout when the sun is high. Use only a slightly less powerful sunscreen if you want to tan. Remember, darker skinned people are better equipped to deal with the sun. If you are particularly fair, choose false tanning creams or eat more beta-carotene! Not only do carotenoids give your skin a coppery shade, but some believe they give you extra protection against the sun.

Remember that no sunscreen offers total protection. They only stop sunburn, which is meant to alarm us to overexposure. Also, while most products block UVB rays, they only minimally block UVA exposure. And UVA rays also contribute to certain skin cancers and accelerate skin aging.

The Good Side of the Sun

The sun has been vilified for many years, but it has an essential purpose. We need sun exposure for vitamin D. Therefore, indulge yourself, but only for thirty minutes a day and with sufficient protection, chosen according to your particular skin type. Never expose your face to the sun. Rather, use a total sunscreen at all times, and wear a hat as often as you can. Antioxidants are added to a number of cosmetic products nowadays, but they cannot combat the effect of UVB rays. Free radicals have a very short life, so your antidote must work the moment free radicals attack your skin. Recently, however, researchers have shown that the flavonoids appearing in grape seeds, pine bark, and green tea are effective against free-radical action. Not surprisingly, when flavonoids are added to cosmetics, they act as strong antioxidants, and protect us from the sun.

Moisturize

To nourish and protect the skin means to combat dehydration. A dry skin is more than dry on the surface, it is depleted of moisture right through the dermis. While moisturized skin is soft and pliable, a dehydrated skin can wrinkle and sag. Whether you are a man or a woman, apply a moisturizing cream every day. Many new treatments include hormones, vitamins, embryo and placenta extracts, and claim to regenerate the skin after damage and aging.

Regenerate Your Skin

The acid vitamin A, tretinoin, popularly known as *Retin-A*, is the only scientifically controlled treatment that acts on the skin's collagen and is proven to regenerate aged, damaged skin. Usually, dermatologists suggest you apply Retin-A every night, or every second night, depending on your skin's tolerance for the treatment. They also insist that you be especially cautious about exposing your face to the sun with this treatment. Though they have no effect on collagen, the action of fruit acids and glycolic acids is reminiscent of acid vitamin A. Their light peeling effect improves your skin's condition.

Treat Superficial Lesions and Wrinkles

Keratosis, brown spots, and other "cemetery flowers" that signify age on your face and hands can also be treated with carbonic snow or laser therapy. Ask your dermatologist about these easy therapies.

In order to eliminate minor imperfections and superficial wrinkles, chemical peels, dermabrasions, and laser applications destroy the top layers of the epidermis. Additionally, laser therapy and chemical peels make your skin retract, which smoothes out minor wrinkles and slightly lifts sagging, particularly around the eyes.

Similarly, collagen injections, or "filling" the wrinkles with fat extracted from your stomach or thighs, can temporarily plump up the deeper lines on your face. None of these therapies replaces a face-lift, but they certainly delay your need for surgery. And after a face-lift, they can help to smooth out any last imperfections.

As you age, the fat in the subcutaneous tissue under the dermis depletes and sinks to the lower part of your face. This is why older faces display hollowed temples and cheeks and also turn "jowly."

Massage

To prevent overdistention of your facial muscles, try deep massages as long as you are careful not to stretch your skin. Also, isometric facial exercises are beneficial but only as long as you do not stretch your skin. Your goal is simply to improve muscle tone, and lift your face naturally, or with the help of electric currents.

Bones

Your facial bones play an integral role in the architecture of your face, and therefore the way you display your age. If you have strong features, prominent bones behind the eyebrows, high cheekbones, a square jaw, and a protruding chin, you are blessed with anchoring points for the flesh of your face, and therefore a reduced tendency to sag.

Unfortunately, if your facial structure is smooth and round, your face droops more readily. If you choose plastic surgery, remember that many facial skeletons are asymmetrical. You may have lived with your personal asymmetry for so long that you are no longer aware of it. That is why plastic surgeons take "before" photographs of their clients' faces, and point out the asymmetry before they begin work. When your appearance changes after surgery, you may suddenly notice the asymmetry and blame it on your doctor! A face-lift cannot correct your basic bone structure.

Bones atrophy and become thinner with age. Even facial bones do. To restore your diminished cheekbones and chin, ask your doctor about coral implants or silicone prostheses. These are rare but effective procedures.

If you have had teeth removed, the gums and gum bones in which your teeth were set will atrophy too. Ask your dentist about dental prostheses where false teeth are inserted into the void. This is a good way to restore roundness to your cheeks.

SMAS

The muscles and the less elastic, fibrous tissue under the subcutaneous layer of the skin merge in a fabriclike network we call *Superficial Musculo-Aponeurotic System*, or SMAS. This tissue and the deeper plane of muscles below it slacken and distend with advancing age. That is how your face sags. When performing a face-lift, a plastic surgeon may focus primarily on the muscle or the skin, depending on which procedure is currently fashionable! Both procedures are effective. Good surgeons ignore fashion and work effectively with both.

Facial Cosmetic Surgery

When we reach forty, our age begins to reveal itself, especially in our faces. Our sagging cheeks accentuate the folds around our nose, our neck slackens, and we see the first signs of a double chin. Now is the time to consider a face-lift.

Sagging eyebrows create a loop in our upper eyelids. Also, crow's feet, small bags under the eyes, as well as some sagging of the lower lids suggest the need for an eye-lift, which is often performed along with a face-lift.

In fact, upper or lower eye-lifts—blepharoplasties—without a face-lift are rarely performed on older people. In eugeria, we follow the dictum of "all or nothing": You must be open to a complete face-lift, which includes work on your eyelids and forehead, or opt to have no work done at all. If you are not 100 percent ready psychologically or financially, hold off on cosmetic surgery until you are ready for a complete procedure. Other treatments, such as collagen injections, will serve you well in the interim.

Having said that, if you do see yourself as a candidate for plastic surgery, try not to delay. Over time, wrinkles settle and their removal becomes even more difficult. Ideally, plastic surgery, like the healthy philosophy that motivates your eugeria, is always preventive rather than curative.

Not that it is ever too late for plastic surgery. You can have your first lift at fifty or sixty and still enjoy good results. But if you undergo your first lift at forty, you will prevent the onset of sagging and give yourself a head start on long-term good looks. Conversely, if you begin at age fifty or sixty, and repeat the procedure every ten years, you will still not enjoy the same effects. Have your first lift at forty, at the very first signs of aging. Never mind that my oldest patient was ninety-one when she had her first lift and had her second at ninety-four! (She told me she was due to see her granddaughters for the first time in years and wanted to clean up the drapey skin around her neck.) *Eugeria* is not a treatise on face-lifts. I have already written that book in French, *From Dream to Reality with Cosmetic*

Surgery (La Table Ronde, 1975). Since then, many reports have been compiled. If you are interested in plastic surgery, I suggest you consult one of them. Though a face-lift is far from life threatening, it is not simple surgery. On the contrary, the operation is a long and meticulous procedure. A face-lift and eye-lift take up to five hours, and lifting the forehead takes about ninety minutes more.

Choosing a Cosmetic Surgeon

Choosing your surgeon will be your most difficult problem. His or her experience must be key to your choice. Contrary to what you read in the press, board certification, or membership in certain scientific societies, does not guarantee skill or experience. Certainly they point to some knowledge, but that is not enough. Keep your ears open for good "word of mouth" testimonials, and keep in mind that certain environments are predisposed to an interest in facial aesthetics. For example, you are likely to hear about good surgeons from satisfied clients in cities like Los Angeles. Let client satisfaction be your ultimate guide. If all else fails, ask your hairdresser! He or she is exposed to a myriad of scars concealed by the hairline and, not surprisingly, is often privy to news about doctors who perform lifts! One more thing: Having chosen a surgeon, know that the technical problems are the doctor's domain. In my experience, many clients are misinformed by brief and shabbily constructed news stories that claim "miracle" procedures or brand-new approaches. A good plastic surgeon keeps abreast of developments and has a far better understanding of various procedures than does the popular press. Further, while new procedures do make their way onto the market periodically, for those in eugeria, I advise against new, experimental approaches. Let others be guinea pigs! And be cautious with all the "mini" or "soft" lifts that are advertised: Predictably, the results are often "mini" as well.

If you learn one thing from this book, let it be the importance of establishing a long-term strategy for a healthy eugeria. This includes cosmetic surgery if you choose it, but cosmetic surgery involves far more than simply scheduling a face-lift at a certain time in your life. You must plan your operations over the long-term to keep your face looking as young as possible, for as long as possible.

Surgical Strategy against Facial Aging

Normally, a good lift will last you ten years. If you were fortunate enough to have your first lift at age forty, then at fifty your face will look as it did ten years before. Since you probably had no work done on your forehead at forty, you will notice it beginning to show signs of sagging. Your eyebrows are lower and a horizontal line has appeared at the root of your nose. Also, due to repeated changes of facial expressions, some deep horizontal lines may now cross your forehead.

Five or six years after your first face-lift is a good time to sched-ule the forehead. This procedure guarantees what we call in French a *coup de jeune*, that is, a shot in the arm, or an instant rejuvena-tor. It lightens the upper part of the face until your next face-lift.

At age fifty you are ready for your second face-lift. Not that the second lift is imperative. On the contrary, you can reap the ben-efits of your first lift for many years. The trouble is, most patients are eager for subsequent lifts. As their surgeon, my job is usually to resist their impatience.

Can You Have Too Many Lifts?

Only a few say: "Here I am, fifty years old, with two major face-lifts under my belt! Isn't there a limit to the number of face-lifts I can endure? I can't carry on like this! I have read that my face will become immobile and drawn!" If ever there was misinfor-mation, this must be it. Your face-lifts must be conducted at reasonable intervals and with expertise. As long as your surgeon undermines your skin and measures the traction to the muscles carefully, there is no limit to the number of lifts you can have.

Pitfalls to Surgery

There is only one major pitfall: Each time a section of your scalp is removed, your hairline recedes. To avoid this, some surgeons make their incisions in front of the hairline during the first lift. To my mind, this is risky: We are never sure how a patient will scar and whether that scar will ever be visible. Therefore, it is best to do this during the second or third lift, when you are left with no other alternative. When the cuts are made in front of the hairline in subsequent lifts, the hairline will move forward and return to its natural position. Clearly, you risk your hairline becoming receded at the temple after one or two excisions in the scalp. This makes for a very odd look. For the forehead, surgeons often make the incision directly in front of the hairline, particularly if your forehead is naturally high. With the removal of skin, your forehead moves up, and your hairline moves down. In the end, your forehead appears smaller.

Second and Third Lifts

You do not need to redo your eyes at your second lift. At best, you may consider work on your double chin and the sagging muscles around your neck. Also, you may consider local collagen shots to smooth out minor wrinkles.

At age sixty, it is time for a major cleanup. In French, we call it a *ravalement*. Your face, forehead, and eyelids must be redone completely. Also, you should consider dermabrasion or laser treatment on your lips. When we get older, our lips are inclined to lengthen and become thinner. To address this, your plastic sur-

geon removes a narrow strip of skin at the border of the vermil-
ion part of the lip. This procedure pulls up the lip to widen the
red surface area and to make it look fuller.

Your First Lift at Age Sixty

If your first lift is at age sixty, consider a second lift after one or two
years. This is because a first lift at this age inevitably leaves a few
imperfections and some secondary sagging often appears. While
neither operation is ever as successful as a first lift at forty, this subsequent lift helps to iron out any remaining or reappearing irregularities. Also, since your nose invariably lengthens with age, now is
the time to schedule a nose job if your aging nose bothers you.

Looking Forty at Sixty

At age sixty, you look like you are forty! What a confidence boost!
You look in the mirror and see no signs of decay. Now are you
ready to accept your eugeria? Will you say, "Enough with cosmetic surgery, I've got a head start, time to age gracefully?" Wish
it were true: So many who begin plastic surgery continually return to their doctors for further help. And while most surgeons
doubt they need extra work, how many refuse their anxious clients?
At best, they can persuade their patients to wait a few years. Of
course, in the world we live in, more women than men become
obsessed with physical perfection. The majority of men I have
treated enjoy their first face- and eye-lift at fifty, their second at
sixty, then leave it at that.

CHAPTER THIRTEEN

Keeping Your Body Young

The same elements rule the body and extremities as do the face: skin, subcutaneous fat tissue, muscles, and bones. The skin on our body suffers the same wear and tear as the skin on our face, except it is less exposed to the sun. However, some women's skin is distended by pregnancy, especially when they put on too much weight before birthing. Distension causes stretch marks, particularly on the breasts and stomach. Likewise, if you have ever been obese and slimmed down dramatically, you may well have stretch marks. On the inside of our arms and legs, our skin is thinner and is more vulnerable to stretching and wrinkles.

FIRM SKIN ON THE BODY

How do we preserve the firm skin on our body? First avoid excessive sun exposure. Second, avoid large fluctuations in weight-gain or loss. However, once you have stretch marks and sagging, there is little you can do about it. You can try creams, physiotherapy, and exercise until you are blue in the face, but the only treatment that works is plastic surgery, especially for the marks on your breasts and abdomen.

Fat Deposits

Fat tissue accumulates in particular areas according to your sex. In women, fat stores appear in the lower abdomen, buttocks, thighs, and the inside of the knees. In men, they are more likely to appear in the upper- and mid-section of the abdomen and the top of the hips, those famous "love handles."

Diet, exercise, massage, and local treatment such as ionization—which sends an electric current into fat stores to dissolve them—or local injections of alphachymotrypsin or hyaluronidase, which diffuse fat deposits, work well in light cases. However, once fat cells are made they remain in the body. This means the buildup of fat will probably reoccur.

Liposuction

Fortunately, liposuction removes fat cells once depleted by diet and exercise that are eagerly waiting to be plumped up again. A canula is inserted into the fat deposits through a tiny incision, and the fat cells are carefully sucked out through the pipe. There is a trade-off for older patients, however: aging skin is no longer elastic, so "wavy" or sagging skin often follows liposuction. When men and women over fifty opt for liposuction, they must also consider a skin resection of the treated area—and this presupposes an unavoidable scar. Here is the cost of cosmetic surgery: the inevitable choice between deformity and scarring. The surgeon's art is to create the best possible shape with the least scarring.

Muscles

Our muscles tend to atrophy and distend as we age. Physical exercise is the best antidote for this. If you are too lazy to lift weight, try excito-motor currents that make the muscles contract and

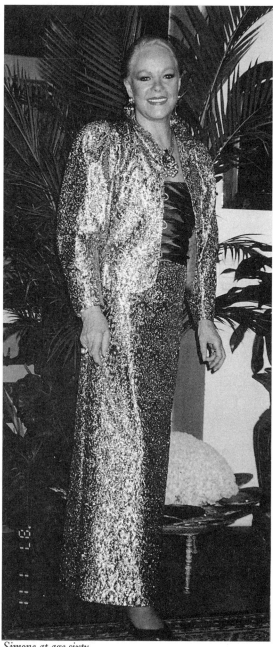

Simone at age sixty

relax. However, you should know that these are no substitute for aerobic activity, which is essential for your general health. Recently there has been some research into administering growth hormones or steroids to rejuvenate muscle and reduce fat deposits. However, these experiments are so new that I do not recommend them to older patients.

Plastic Surgery of the Body

Plastic surgery of the body is most often directed toward significant deformities of the breasts and stomach. After age fifty, most people learn to accept their small or droopy breasts, or their slight paunch. However, there is no reason for you to live with heavy, uncomfortable, and sagging breasts or a stomach that falls to your thighs like an apron.

Mammoplasty

Mammoplasty reduces the mammary glands in your breasts and also dispenses excess skin. Part of the remaining skin is redraped over your reduced glands, so your nipples are transposed to a higher position. At first, reduced breasts assume a conical shape, but ultimately round out by the weight of gravity. While there are long scars associated with this procedure, they rarely become red or raised in older people. More often than not they fade altogether. Interestingly, old people don't make as much scar tissue as their young counterparts. They just don't have the collagen to build up the scar tissue.

Abdominoplasty

When your plastic surgeon performs abdominoplasty, or tummy tuck, he cuts along the fold above the pubis, extending from the top of one hip to the other. Your skin, subcutaneous tissue, and fat are pulled—undermined—from the fibrous layer above the muscles, and from the initial incision up to the rib cage. A liposuction

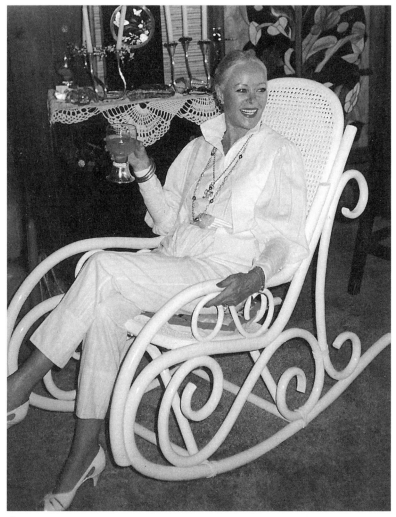

Simone at age sixty-nine

procedure removes excess fat from the upper part of the stomach. Next the surgeon applies a tuck to the aponeurosis and the muscles in order to tighten the abdominal wall. The excess skin and fat tissue floating below the navel are removed and discarded. Then the surgeon sews up the wound, and your belly button, which was left attached to the deep structure of the abdomen, is retrieved per incision and sewn to the lips of the new skin around it.

Wrinkles Inside the Arms and Thighs
Though it is difficult to accept, the older you get, the more your skin becomes distended, especially where it is thinnest. This is why it wrinkles on the inside of your arms and thighs. Though these areas most accurately reveal your age, a simple removal of the excess skin solves your problem in minutes. Slim individuals are even more prone to sagging skin. If overall sagging skin is a problem, ask your surgeon about excising a several centimeters wide strip of skin all around the body at the level of the submammary fold or the scar of the mammoplasty. This is not a common operation but most patients are satisfied with it.

SIMONE

Here are some of my thoughts on preventing as much as possible the aging of the face and the body:
I maintain a proper diet with food supplements and antioxidants. I abstain from smoking and drinking too much alcohol, and avoid exposure to the sun. These are common well-known recommendations, but I want to insist on the necessity of maintaining a good level of hormones, especially of estrogen. It is surprising to see and I have observed it closely on others how the skin becomes dehydrated and deep wrinkles can appear in one year after menopause. I am sure that the quality of my skin, which has kept its tone and thickness at seventy-four, is in great part due to the estrogen treatment I have received during the past forty-eight years.
Besides these general measures against skin aging, specific skin care is equally important to protect and regenerate the skin. Since the face is the most exposed to the aging factors, it is the one that should benefit most from skin care. I am willing to give you the details of the skin treatment I generally use at night and in the morning. The selection is the result of trying

many of the best-known products. But, be warned, there are many types of skin; mine is rather thick and on the greasy side. What works for me will not necessarily give the same result for your skin type.

Skin Treatment for the Night

Before going to bed I thoroughly clean my face with a special liquid soap or cleansing milk. With a clean sponge, I remove all traces of makeup from my face and neck. At least three times a week I apply Retin-A, massaging lightly to make it penetrate the skin. The other days of the week I use an antiaging or antioxidant cream on my face, neck, and the exposed part of the décolleté. I also use the cream on the back of my hands, and instead of wiping my hands on a towel (which certainly does not need my precious cream), I wipe the excess off on my arms.

Skin Treatment for the Day

If the treatment for the night is especially designed to regenerate the skin, the treatment for the day is more oriented to its protection and appearance. Makeup is a must for anyone who has some interest in appearance (even more so after cosmetic surgery where there might be some scars to camouflage). There is no doubt that your makeup will be different based upon your skin type and the area where you live. In a cold, windy area or in very dry climate, the skin needs more hydrating and more fat. In California, I generally use as a foundation a Japanese product, which is tinted in gold and is best adapted to my skin (Sammimore, a gold milky-type emollient foundation imported by Jacqui's Corporation, Honolulu).

I have used this product for several years, but I am sorry to say that I have not found its equivalent here or in Europe. Over this foundation I apply makeup, which I try to keep discreet. Some powder if the temperature is hot, to avoid the shine on my nose and my forehead. I use blush on the cheeks, which is often neglected but gives a healthy appearance and brings out the beauty of the eyes. On the eyelids I apply soft-pressed eye shadow that is slightly tinted according to the color of the eyes. I use black mascara for the eyelashes; I am against blue or green mascara, which looks too artificial. To contour my lips, I design with a pencil and fill it with lipstick of very classic color (close to nature—not fancy).

As for the back of my hands (which might betray one's age with black spots, dilated veins, and wrinkles), I use the same Japanese foundation, and when I drive I wear gloves to protect my hands from the sun.

Whatever skin care you use will help but not prevent the sagging and the wrinkles of the skin. This is where cosmetic surgery will help. As for myself, I have followed the plan advocated by my husband and had my first face-lift and eyelid operation at the age of forty. I have had several since and just before sending the completed book to our publisher, while on our vacation in France, I had the opportunity to have my husband and his pupil and friend Dr. Bernard Candon do a little work on my forehead again. Needless to say, I am very satisfied with the result.

Why I Believe in Eugeria

Too many aging people, thinking they are doing the right thing, embark on diets or take supplements haphazardly depending on circumstances or publicity without knowing exactly what they are taking or at what dose. Certain components make double use and others are lacking completely, which can lead to serious imbalances, and this is not without risk.

In this book I have tried to establish a program including all the positive things you can do to promote a healthy and active old age, what I have called *eugeria*. First of all, you must accept the idea of aging, because it is not by denying it but by facing it with all your determination and willpower that you will succeed in prolonging your eugeria until the genetically programmed end. Unless future gene manipulations make us immortal, death should also be prepared for. But it would be the subject of another book.

It is up to you to decide what efforts or sacrifices you are ready to make in order to live better and longer. I have not insisted here on the most arduous path toward longevity, and unless you have real faith in a discipline such as Dr. Walford's diet, do not attempt to so radically change your lifestyle. In fact, for other lazy souls like me, the most difficult step in attaining eugeria will probably be making sure you perform a minimum amount of exercise every day.

The program I have outlined for you is based on scientific studies, which are the most reliable sources of information. Even though medicine is not an exact science, when a kind of consensus appears to have been reached, we can usually trust the validity of the result. Even the longest and the most reliable studies, like the

Framingham study, can be at fault because some factors were unknown at the time they were started (cholesterol for example was condemned but homocysteine was ignored).

I am not a twentieth century Dr. Faust with a magic potion (not even the antioxidants fit this definition), nor am I the reincarnation of Ponce de Leon. There is no "fountain of youth" dispensing an elixir that will eliminate the necessity of your making your own effort towards attaining eugeria.

To my eyes, the most significant proof of the success of my program is the dramatic impact it has had on my own life and on that of my wife, Simone.

I know it has no scientific value, nevertheless maybe you would like to hear our story.

MY CASE

My own genetic heritage could not have been worse. Both my parents died of vascular problems, my mother at sixty-three of stroke, my father at seventy-two with cerebral vascular infarcts.

At forty I was very absorbed in my work as a plastic surgeon and found myself smoking about thirty cigarettes a day and exercising only rarely. When I began to have chest pains I made an appointment with the cardiologist and the results were not encouraging: the electrocardiogram showed signs of some coronary insufficiency, my blood pressure was at 160, there were high lipids in my blood, and my cholesterol was over 4 g per liter. In other words, at the age of forty I was a prime candidate for a heart attack.

What to do? I stopped smoking and went on a diet to lose some twenty pounds. I was treated for high cholesterol and put on beta-blockers. My cholesterol did go down but my triglycerides remained high, and I still had some chest pain occasionally.

By the time I was sixty, the prospect of a long, healthy old age was slightly better than it had been twenty years earlier, but I certainly was not in a state of eugeria. (In fact, one of my doctor "friends" warned prospective clients to choose another surgeon since I might very well drop dead during the operation.)

It was time to really get serious about the next twenty (or more if I was lucky) years of my existence. To begin I moved from Paris to Tahiti for a change of life and a less heavy schedule. And then I started on my program for eugeria: Watching my diet, eating lots of raw fish, taking multivitamins, multiminerals, and antioxidants, seriously endeavoring to overcome my natural laziness by swimming every day in the pool. I continued at the same time to take my medication for high cholesterol, high blood pressure, and coronary insufficiency. Subsequently, my blood pressure stabilized around 140 and my chest pain under stress was less than it had been for years.

Since I began this regimen, eighteen years have elapsed. For the past three years I have taken aspirin (330 mg every other day) and I practice tai chi about half an hour a day. I can read the newspaper without glasses (although I use them to work), and my hearing (which was beginning to fail) has now stabilized. As for my brain? It is still working pretty well, thank you!

Over my lifetime I have had three face-lift and eye-lift operations at ages fifty-two, sixty-three, and seventy-four, which have prevented me from having the sagging face and baggy eyelids that were already making their appearance shortly after my fiftieth birthday.

And my retirement at the beginning of 1997 was not due to my feeling I could not still operate at my best, but for family reasons I will explain later, and also because I was tired of fighting against the discrimination faced by many elderly professionals who are being forced from their position solely because of their age. In addition, since 1993, I have been fighting (pretty successfully so far) prostate cancer with multiple bone metastases, in spite of which I still consider myself living in the best mental and physical eugeria possible under the circumstances.

SIMONE'S CASE

As for my wife, Simone, after forty-five years of cloudless marriage (which is by itself an important factor for attaining eugeria
and longevity), and although she has reached the respectable age
of seventy-four, her activity level and her appearance (as you can
judge from the photographs in this book) would never betray
her years. As in my own case, Simone had early bad experiences,
which were an obstacle to eugeria. Her father died at forty-eight
of an accident and her mother at forty of cancer. She had a son
from her first marriage, whose birth by caesarean was followed by
complications which necessitated a hysterectomy and ovariectomy
at age nineteen. This operation caused many health problems due
to hormonal deprivation which continued until she began replacement hormone treatment ten years later in the form of estrogen pellets that were inserted under the skin and lasted about
two years. Ten years ago these hormone pellets disappeared from
the French pharmacopeia apparently for marketing reasons, since
they were ideal for women with hysterectomies. Since then she
has been using injections every month, and later patches, and now
a gel. She continues using this therapy both to fight aging, and
also because, as soon as the treatment is interrupted, the deprivation symptoms return. Since she was thirty-five, Simone has also
suffered from osteoarthritis, mainly in the spine, and has undergone a diversity of treatments from doctors, chiropractors, and
osteopaths with varying degrees of success. The one prescription,
however, which she can always rely on is aspirin (330 mg daily,
even 500 mg when she is in pain).

Although it didn't prevent the recent formation of nodules on
her fingers (which, of course, she hates), she claims her life has
changed since she started her aspirin therapy. For the last eighteen
years we have pursued together the eugeria program I have outlined here (including the red wine, which she appreciates), and I
am inclined to measure the program's success in terms of, among
other things, her indomitable energy and unquenchable zest for

life. In fact, it was these attributes which led us twelve years ago to adopt a little Tahitian girl who has, since her birth, been entirely in Simone's care. At the age of seventy-four, my wife drives Daisy to and from school and to dancing and piano lessons. She supervises her homework and is even being initiated into the mystic realm of "modern" mathematics. It was mostly for Daisy's sake that we moved to Los Angeles, where she is now in eighth grade at the Lycee Français and on her way to becoming fluently bilingual. Actually, if a metaphorical fountain of youth does exist, it may well be found in the company of children. To be responsible for the care of a child, for that child's physical and emotional needs, for the education of her mind and heart can be a tremendously rejuvenating experience; the concern about her future is also a positive encouragement to survive in eugeria as long as possible. Besides being a "young" mother, Simone is also a typical example of "looking" young. She knew how to take care of her skin and protect it from the sun. She has exhausted all the resources of cosmetic surgery against aging, although fortunately she didn't need any corrective surgery at the start. She had her first face-lift (and eyelids) done at age forty, a second facelift (without the eyes) at fifty, a third face-lift with the eyelids and the forehead at fifty-eight, and a fourth face-lift (in front of the hairline) at sixty-seven. I must say she is a perfectionist who does not tolerate any flaws, and she does have at hand a surgeon who cannot refuse her any operation.

On her body she has undergone all the cosmetic operations you can imagine, with the ransom of some discreet scars that she prefers (me too) to the sagging of old age. Considering her present state of health and energy, unless an unforeseen event intervenes, I think she will enjoy a long and active eugeria.

I very well know that our stories are no scientific proof of the efficacy of my program, but they are living examples of people who were not especially predisposed to attaining and maintaining eugeria. If you are ready to follow Simone in her quest for a youthful appearance and a life-full old age, I can not guarantee but I can reasonably wish you a happy and prolonged eugeria.

Nutritive Value of Food

Dairy Products

	Measure	Grams	Calories	Protein (Grams)	Fat (Grams)	Saturated Fat (Grams)	Carbohydrate (Grams)	Calcium (milligrams)	Iron (milligrams)	Sodium (milligrams)	Vitamin A (I.U.)	Ascorbic Acid (milligrams)
Cheese, cheddar, cut pieces	1 oz.	28	115	7	9	6.0	T	204	0.2	176	300	0
Cheese, cottage, small curd	1 cup	210	215	26	9	6.0	6	126	0.3	850	340	T
Cheese, cream	1 oz.	28	100	2	10	6.2	1	23	0.3	84	400	0
Cheese, Swiss	1 oz.	28	95	7	7	4.5	1	219	0.2	388	230	0
Half-and-half	1 tbsp.	15	20	T	2	1.1	1	16	T	6	70	T
Cream, sour	1 tbsp.	12	25	T	3	1.6	1	14	T	6	90	T
Milk, whole	1 cup	244	150	8	8	5.1	11	291	0.1	120	310	2
Milk, nonfat (skim)	1 cup	245	85	8	T	0.3	12	302	0.1	126	500	2
Milkshake, chocolate	10 oz.	283	355	9	8	4.8	60	374	0.9	314	240	0
Ice cream, hardened	1 cup	133	270	5	14	8.9	32	176	0.1	116	540	1
Sherbet	1 cup	193	270	2	4	2.4	59	103	0.3	88	190	4
Yogurt, fruit-flavored	8 oz.	227	230	10	2	1.6	43	345	0.2	133	100	1

T = trace;

‡ = value not determined.

Note: Values shown here for these foods may be from several different manufacturers and, therefore, may differ somewhat from the values provided by a single source.

Source: Home and Garden Bulletin No. 72; U.S. Dept. of Agriculture.

	Measure	Grams	Calories	Protein (Grams)	Fat (Grams)	Saturated Fat (Grams)	Carbohydrate (Grams)	Calcium (milligrams)	Iron (milligrams)	Sodium (milligrams)	Vitamin A (I.U.)	Ascorbic Acid (milligrams)
Eggs												
Fried in margarine	1	46	90	6	7	1.9	1	25	0.7	162	390	0
Hard-cooked	1	50	75	6	5	1.6	1	25	0.6	62	280	0
Scrambled (milk added) in margarine	1	61	100	7	7	2.2	1	44	0.7	171	420	T
Fats & oils												
Butter, salted	1 tbsp.	14	100	T	11	7.1	T	3	T	116	430	0
Margarine, salted	1 tbsp.	14	100	T	11	2.2	T	4	T	132	460	T
Olive oil	1 tbsp.	14	125	0	14	1.9	0	0	0	0	0	0
Salad dressing, blue cheese	1 tbsp.	15	75	1	8	1.5	1	12	T	164	30	T
Salad dressing, French, regular	1 tbsp.	16	85	T	9	1.4	1	2	T	188	T	T
Salad dressing, French, lo-cal	1 tbsp.	16	25	T	2	0.2	2	6	T	306	T	T
Salad dressing, Italian	1 tbsp.	15	80	T	9	1.3	1	1	T	162	30	T
Mayonnaise	1 tbsp.	14	100	T	11	1.7	T	3	0.1	80	40	0
Fish, meat, poultry												
Clams, raw, meat only	3 oz.	85	65	11	1	0.3	2	59	2.6	102	90	9
Crabmeat, canned	1 cup	135	135	23	3	0.5	1	61	1.1	1,350	50	0
Fish sticks, frozen, reheated	1 fish stick	28	70	6	3	0.8	4	11	0.3	53	20	0
Salmon canned (pink), solids and liquid	3 oz.	85	120	17	5	0.9	0	167	0.7	443	60	0

Food	Portion											
Sardines, Atlantic, canned in oil, drained solids	3 oz.	85	175	20	9	2.1	0	371	2.6	425	190	0
Shrimp, French fried	3 oz.	85	200	16	10	2.5	11	61	2.0	384	90	0
Trout, broiled, with butter and lemon juice	3 oz.	85	175	21	9	4.1	T	26	1.0	122	230	1
Tuna, canned in oil	3 oz.	85	165	24	7	1.4	0	7	1.6	303	70	0
Bacon, broiled or fried crisp	3 slices	19	110	6	9	3.3	T	2	0.3	303	0	6
Ground beef, broiled, regular	3 oz.	85	245	20	18	6.9	0	9	2.1	70	T	0
Roast beef, relatively lean (lean only)	2.6 oz.	75	135	22	5	1.9	0	3	1.5	46	T	0
Beef steak, lean and fat	3 oz.	85	240	23	15	6.4	0	9	2.6	53	T	0
Beef & vegetable stew	1 cup	245	220	16	11	4.4	15	29	2.9	292	5,690	17
Lamb, chop, broiled loin, lean and fat	2.8 oz.	80	235	22	16	7.3	0	16	1.4	62	T	0
Liver, beef, fried	3 oz.	85	185	23	7	2.5	7	9	5.3	90	30,690	23
Ham, light cure, roasted, lean and fat	3 oz.	85	205	18	14	5.1	0	6	0.7	1,009	0	0
Pork, chop, broiled, lean and fat	3.1 oz.	87	275	24	19	7.0	0	3	0.7	61	10	T
Bologna	2 slices	57	180	7	16	6.1	2	7	0.9	581	0	12
Frankfurter, pork, cooked	1	45	145	5	13	4.8	1	5	0.5	504	0	12
Sausage, pork link, cooked	1 link	13	50	3	4	1.4	T	4	0.2	168	0	T
Veal, cutlet, braised or broiled	3 oz.	85	185	23	9	4.1	0	9	0.8	56	T	0
Chicken, drumstick, fried, bones removed	2.5 oz.	72	195	16	11	3.0	6	12	1.0	194	60	0
Chicken, roasted, half breast, without skin	3 oz.	86	140	27	3	0.9	0	13	0.9	64	20	0

	Grams	Calories	Protein (Grams)	Fat (Grams)	Saturated Fat (Grams)	Carbohydrate (Grams)	Calcium (milligrams)	Iron (milligrams)	Sodium (milligrams)	Vitamin A (I.U.)	Ascorbic Acid (milligrams)
Turkey, roasted, chopped light and dark meat	1 cup	140	240	41	7	2.3	0	35	2.5	98	0	0
Frankfurter, chicken, cooked	1	45	115	6	9	2.5	3	43	0.9	616	60	0
Fruits & fruit products											
Apple, raw, 2¾ in. diam	1	138	80	T	T	0.1	21	10	0.2	T	70	8
Apple juice	1 cup	248	115	T	T	T	29	17	0.9	7	T	2
Apricots, raw	3	106	50	1	T	T	12	15	0.6	1	2,770	11
Banana, raw	1	114	105	1	1	0.2	27	7	0.4	1	90	10
Cherries, sweet, raw	10	68	50	1	T	0.1	11	10	0.3	T	150	5
Cranberry juice, sweetened	1 cup	253	145	T	T	T	38	8	0.4	10	10	108
Fruit cocktail, canned, in heavy syrup	1 cup	255	185	1	T	T	48	15	0.7	15	520	5
Grapefruit, raw, med., white	½	120	40	1	T	T	10	14	0.1	T	10	41
Grapes, Thompson seedless	10	50	35	T	T	0.1	9	6	0.1	1	40	5
Lemonade, frozen, unsweetened	6 oz.	244	55	1	1	0.1	16	20	0.3	2	30	77
Cantaloupe, 5-in. diam	½	267	95	2	1	0.1	22	29	0.6	24	8,610	113
Orange, 2⅝ in. diam	1	131	60	1	T	T	15	52	0.1	T	270	70
Orange juice, frozen, diluted	1 cup	249	110	2	T	T	27	22	0.2	2	190	97
Peach, raw, 2½ in. diam	1	87	35	1	T	T	10	4	0.1	T	470	6

Food	Measure	Weight (g)	Calories	Protein	Fat	Sat. fat	Carbohydrate	Calcium	Iron	Sodium	Vitamin A	Vitamin C
Raisins, seedless	1 cup	145	435	5	1	0.2	115	71	3.0	17	10	5
Strawberries, whole	1 cup	149	45	1	1	T	10	21	0.6	1	40	84
Watermelon, 4 × 8 in. wedge	1 piece	482	155	3	2	0.3	35	39	0.8	10	1,760	46
Grain Products												
Bagel, plain	1	68	200	7	2	0.3	38	29	1.8	245	0	0
Biscuit, 2 in. diam., from home recipe	1	28	100	2	5	1.2	13	47	0.7	195	10	T
Bread, pita, enriched, white, 6½ in. diam	1 pita	60	165	6	1	0.1	12	15	0.7	124	0	0
Bread, white, enriched	1 slice	25	65	2	1	0.3	12	32	0.7	129	T	T
Bread, whole-wheat	1 slice	28	70	3	1	0.4	13	20	1.0	150	T	T
Oatmeal or rolled oats, without added salt	1 cup	234	145	6	2	0.4	25	19	1.6	2	40	0
Bran flakes (40% bran), added sugar, salt, iron, vitamins	1 oz.	28	90	4	1	0.1	22	14	8.1	264	1,250	0
Corn flakes, added sugar, salt, iron, vitamins	1 oz.	28	110	2	T	T	24	1	1.8	351	1,250	15
Rice, puffed, added iron, thiamine, niacin	1 oz.	28	110	2	T	T	25	4	1.8	340	1,250	15
Wheat, shredded, plain, 1 biscuit or ⅔ cup	1 oz.	28	100	3	1	0.1	23	11	1.2	3	0	0
Bulgur, uncooked	1 cup	170	600	19	3	1.2	129	49	9.5	7	0	0
Cake, angel food, ½ slice	1	53	125	3	T	T	29	44	0.2	269	0	0
Cupcake, 2½ in. diam., with chocolate icing	1	35	120	2	4	1.8	20	21	0.7	92	50	T

	Measure	Grams	Calories	Protein (Grams)	Fat (Grams)	Saturated Fat (Grams)	Carbohydrate (Grams)	Calcium (milligrams)	Iron (milligrams)	Sodium (milligrams)	Vitamin A (I.U.)	Ascorbic Acid (milligrams)
Plain sheet cake with white, uncooked frosting, ⅑ slice	1	121	445	4	14	4.6	77	61	1.2	275	240	T
Fruitcake, dark, ½₀ of loaf	1	43	165	2	7	1.5	25	41	1.2	67	50	16
Cake, pound, ½₇ of loaf	1	29	110	2	5	3.0	15	8	0.5	108	160	0
Cheesecake, ½₂ of 9-in. cake	1	92	280	5	18	9.9	26	52	0.4	204	230	5
Brownies, with nuts, from commercial recipe	1	25	100	1	4	1.6	16	13	0.6	59	70	T
Cookies, chocolate chip, from home recipe	4	40	185	2	11	3.9	26	13	1.0	82	20	0
Crackers, graham, 2½ in. squares	2	14	60	1	1	0.4	11	6	0.4	86	0	0
Crackers, saltines	4	12	50	1	1	0.5	9	3	0.5	165	0	0
Danish pastry, round piece	1	57	220	4	12	3.6	26	60	1.1	218	60	T
Doughnut, cake type	1	50	210	3	12	2.8	24	22	1.0	192	20	T
Macaroni, firm stage (hot)	1 cup	130	190	7	1	0.1	39	14	2.1	1	0	0
Muffin, bran, commercial mix	1	45	140	3	4	1.3	24	27	1.7	385	100	0
Muffin, corn, from home recipe	1	45	145	3	5	1.5	21	66	0.9	169	80	T
Noodles, enriched, cooked	1 cup	160	200	7	2	0.5	37	16	2.6	3	110	0
Pie, apple, ⅙ of pie	1	158	405	3	18	4.6	60	13	1.6	476	50	2
Pie, cherry, ⅙ of pie	1	158	410	4	18	4.7	61	22	1.6	480	700	0

Food	Amount											
Pie, lemon meringue, ⅙ of pie	1	140	355	5	14	4.3	53	20	1.4	395	240	4
Pie, pecan, ⅙ of pie	1	138	575	7	32	4.7	71	65	4.6	305	220	0
Popcorn, air-popped, plain	1 cup	8	30	1	T	T	6	1	0.2	T	10	0
Pretzels, stick	10	3	10	T	T	T	2	1	0.1	48	0	0
Rolls, enriched, brown & serve	1	28	85	2	2	0.5	14	33	0.8	155	T	T
Rolls, frankfurter & hamburger	1	40	115	3	2	0.5	20	54	1.2	241	T	T
Tortillas, corn	1	30	65	2	1	0.1	13	42	0.6	1	80	0

Legumes, Nuts, Seeds

Food	Amount											
Beans, Black	1 cup	171	225	15	1	0.1	41	47	2.9	1	T	0
Beans, Great Northern, cooked	1 cup	180	210	14	1	0.1	38	90	4.9	13	0	0
Peanuts, roasted in oil, salted	1 cup	145	840	39	71	9.9	27	125	2.8	626	0	0
Peanut butter	1 tbsp.	16	95	5	8	1.4	3	5	0.3	75	0	0
Refried beans, canned	1 cup	290	295	18	3	0.4	51	141	5.1	1,228	0	17
Tofu	1 piece	120	85	9	5	0.7	3	108	2.3	8	0	0
Sunflower seeds, hulled	1 oz.	28	160	6	14	1.5	5	33	1.9	1	10	T

Mixed Foods

Food	Amount											
Chop suey with beef and pork, home recipe	1 cup	250	300	26	17	4.3	13	60	4.8	1,053	600	33
Enchilada	1	230	235	20	16	7.7	24	97	3.3	1,332	2,720	T
Pizza, cheese, ⅛ of 15 in.-diam. pie	1	120	290	15	9	4.1	39	220	1.6	699	750	2
Spaghetti with meatballs & tomato sauce	1 cup	248	330	19	12	3.9	39	124	3.7	1,009	1,590	22

Sugars & Sweets

Food	Amount											
Candy, caramels	1 oz.	28	115	1	3	2.2	22	42	0.4	64	T	T

	Measure	Grams	Calories	Protein (Grams)	Fat (Grams)	Saturated Fat (Grams)	Carbohydrate (Grams)	Calcium (milligrams)	Iron (milligrams)	Sodium (milligrams)	Vitamin A (I.U.)	Ascorbic Acid (milligrams)
Candy, milk chocolate	1 oz.	28	145	2	9	5.4	16	50	0.4	23	30	T
Fudge, chocolate	1 oz.	28	115	1	3	2.1	21	22	0.3	54	T	T
Gelatin dessert, from prepared powder	½ cup	120	70	2	0	0.0	17	2	T	55	0	0
Candy, hard	1 oz.	28	110	0	0	0.0	28	T	0.1	7	0	0
Honey	1 tbsp.	21	65	T	0	0.0	17	1	0.1	1	0	T
Jams & Preserves	1 tbsp.	20	55	T	T	0.0	14	4	0.2	2	0	T
Popsicle, 3 fl. oz.	1	95	70	0	0	0.0	18	0	T	11	0	0
Sugar, white, granulated	1 tbsp.	12	45	0	0	0.0	12	T	T	T	0	0

Vegetables

	Measure	Grams	Calories	Protein (Grams)	Fat (Grams)	Saturated Fat (Grams)	Carbohydrate (Grams)	Calcium (milligrams)	Iron (milligrams)	Sodium (milligrams)	Vitamin A (I.U.)	Ascorbic Acid (milligrams)
Asparagus, spears, cooked from raw	4 spears	60	15	2	T	T	3	14	0.4	2	500	16
Beans, green, from frozen, cuts	1 cup	135	35	2	T	T	8	61	1.1	18	710	11
Broccoli, cooked from raw	1 spear	180	50	5	1	0.1	10	82	2.1	20	2,540	113
Cabbage, raw, coarsely shredded or sliced	1 cup	70	15	1	T	T	4	33	0.4	13	90	33
Carrots, raw, 7½ by 1⅛ in.	1	72	30	1	T	T	7	19	0.4	25	20,250	7
Cauliflower, cooked, drained, from raw	1 cup	125	30	2	T	T	6	34	0.5	8	20	69
Celery, raw	1 stalk	40	5	T	T	T	1	14	0.2	35	50	3

Food	Amount											
Collards, cooked from raw	1 cup	190	25	2	T	0.1	5	148	0.8	36	4,220	19
Corn, sweet, yellow, cooked from raw	1 ear	77	85	3	1	0.2	19	2	0.5	13	170	5
Eggplant, cooked, steamed	1 cup	96	25	1	T	T	6	6	0.3	3	60	1
Lettuce, iceberg, chopped	1 cup	55	5	1	T	T	1	10	0.3	5	180	2
Lettuce, looseleaf (such as romaine)	1 cup	56	10	1	T	T	2	38	0.8	5	1,060	10
Mushrooms, raw	1 cup	70	20	1	T	T	3	4	0.9	3	0	2
Onions, raw, chopped	1 cup	160	55	2	T	0.1	12	40	0.6	3	0	13
Peas, green, frozen, cooked	1 cup	160	125	8	T	0.1	23	38	2.5	139	1,070	16
Potatoes, baked, peeled	1	156	145	3	T	T	34	8	0.5	8	0	20
Potatoes, frozen, French fried (oven-heated)	10	50	110	2	4	2.1	17	5	0.7	16	0	5
Potatoes, mashed, milk added	1 cup	210	160	4	1	0.7	37	55	0.6	636	40	14
Potato chips	10	20	105	1	7	1.8	10	5	0.2	94	0	8
Potato salad	1 cup	250	360	7	21	3.6	28	48	1.6	1,323	520	25
Spinach, drained, cooked from raw	1 cup	180	40	5	T	0.1	7	245	6.4	126	14,740	18
Sweet potatoes, baked in skin, peeled	1	114	115	2	T	T	28	32	0.5	11	24,880	28
Tomatoes, raw	1	123	25	1	T	T	5	9	0.6	10	1,390	22
Vegetable juice cocktail, canned	1 cup	242	45	2	T	T	11	27	1.0	883	2,830	67
Miscellaneous												
Beer, regular	12 fl. oz.	360	150	1	0	0.0	13	14	0.1	18	0	0

	Measure	Grams	Calories	Protein (Grams)	Fat (Grams)	Saturated Fat (Grams)	Carbohydrate (Grams)	Calcium (milligrams)	Iron (milligrams)	Sodium (milligrams)	Vitamin A (I.U.)	Ascorbic Acid (milligrams)
Gin, rum, vodka, whisky, 86 proof	1½ fl. oz.	42	105	0	0	0.0	T	T	T	T	0	0
Wine, table, white	3½ fl. oz.	102	80	T	0	0.0	3	9	0.3	5	T	0
Cola-type beverage	12 fl. oz.	369	160	0	0	0.0	41	11	0.2	18	0	0
Ginger ale	12 fl. oz	366	125	0	0	0.0	32	11	0.1	29	0	0
Coffee , brewed	6 fl. oz.	180	T	T	T	T	T	4	T	2	0	0
Tea, brewed	8 fl. oz.	240	T	T	T	T	T	0	T	1	0	0
Catsup	1 tbsp.	15	15	T	T	T	4	3	0.1	156	210	2
Mustard, prepared, yellow	1 tsp.	5	5	T	T	T	T	4	0.1	63	0	T
Olives, canned, green	4 medium	13	15	T	2	0.2	T	8	0.2	312	40	0
Pickles, dill, whole	1	65	5	T	T	T	1	17	0.7	928	70	4
Relish, finely chopped, sweet	1 tbsp.	15	20	T	T	T	5	3	0.1	107	20	1
Soup, tomato, prepared with milk	1 cup	248	160	6	6	2.9	22	159	1.8	932	850	68
Soup, chicken noodle, prepared with water	1 cup	241	75	4	2	0.7	9	17	0.8	1,106	710	T
Soup, green pea, prepared with water	1 cup	250	165	9	3	1.4	27	28	2.0	988	200	2
Soup, vegetarian prepared with water	1 cup	241	70	2	2	0.3	12	22	1.1	822	3,010	1

Index

abdominoplasty, 221–222
accidents, 23, 30–31
acetylcholine, 101, 117
acidophilus, 140
acupuncture, for quitting smoking, 39
adipose tissue, 62–63
adrenaline, 63
age
  causes of death and, 23–24
  face-lifts and, 213–214
aging
  body temperature and, 13
  catastrophic errors in genetic code and, 10
  Denkla's hormonal theory of, 11–12
  free-radical theory of, 10–11
  genetic clock and, 9
  lifestyle adjustments and, 3
  reduced calorie program and, 13
  theories of, 9–14
aging well. *See* eugeria
alcohol consumption, 31, 35, 39–43, 71, 125, 130, 142–145
  recommended intake, 144
alcoholism, 40–43, 41–42, 144–145
algae, 17 8, 61, 139
allicin, 138
Alzheimer's disease, 37, 97, 101, 117, 122, 166
amino acids, essential, 57, 58
  supplements, 160–161
anemia
  macrocytic, 113
  megaloblastic, 110
antioncogenes, 122–123

antioxidants, 92–93, 152–160, 158, 195
  benefits of, 156–157
  cholesterol and, 66
  deactivation by free radicals, 10–11
  endogenous, 153–154
  exogenous, 154–155
  recommended intake, 157–158
  research studies, 157
appearance, importance of, 203–204
arginin, 189
arthritis, 152, 185, 228
Aslan, Anna, 6, 166
aspirin, 184–187, 196, 227, 228
atherosclerosis, 64–66, 65, 66, 120, 163, 174, 181
attention loss, 166

Baulieu, E.-E., 189, 190
bearing, young, 203
beta-blockers, 44, 158, 174
beta-carotene, 92–93, 94, 154, 195
blood pressure, 119. *See also* hypertension
  low, 120
  testing, 25–26
blood-pressure monitors, 26
blood tests, 27
body
  preserving, 219–224, 229
  tuning into, 27
body temperature, 13
body weight. *See* weight
body weight mass index (BMI), 48
bone density tests, 180
brain aging, 161–162

mental activity and, 171–173
prevention of, 162
treating with drugs, 165–166
breast cancer, 28, 182–183
breathing, 169
Brown, Michael S., 66

calcium, 75–77, 95, 151, 195
Calment, Jeanne, 1, 2, 5–6, 15, 156
caloric intake, 51, 135
cancers, 23, 24, 25, 121, 122, 143,
    182, 186
    of colon, 56
    detection of, 24, 25
    genetic-based treatments for,
      123
    oncogenes and, 122–123
    risk factors for, 30
    tobacco and, 36
carbohydrates, 52–55
    recommended intake, 53, 136
cardiovascular disease, 23, 24, 31
    exams for, 27
    risk factors, 30
carotenoids, 92–93, 138, 154–155
catalase, 11, 154
cell(s)
    division of, and aging, 9
    sudden flaws in, and aging, 10
cell membranes, 10, 60
cell therapy, 6, 125, 193–194
cellulase, 55
cellulose, 55–56
centenarians. *See* Calment,
    Jeanne
children, 229
chi qong, 169
chlorine, 74–75
chocolate, 144
cholesterol levels, 30, 60
    atherosclerosis and, 64–65
    fiber and, 56
    garlic and, 148
    genetic factors and, 69

heart attack and, 64, 119
    low, 70–71
    niacin and, 105
    obesity and, 49
    sources of, 66–67, 68
    stress and, 69
choline, 116–117
chromium, 83–84, 136, 151
cloning, 122
coenzyme Q10, 126, 156, 158, 196
collagen, 205
collagen injections, 211, 217
colon cancer, 56
colon cancer, and aspirin, 186
colonoscopies, 25
computers, using, 171–172
copper, 81, 86
cortisone, 105
cosmetic surgery, facial, 212,
    213–218
cruciferous vegetables, 138
cysteine, 155

dairy products, 140
dancing, 173
death
    alcoholic intoxication and, 41
    causes of, in industrialized
      countries, 23–25
DECO, 11–12
De Gennes, 65
Denkla, 11–12
dental exams, 27–28
depression, 130, 163
DHEA, 12, 189, 190, 191, 196
diabetes, 30, 40, 49, 53–55, 84,
    136, 145
diet. *See* nutrition
diseases, infectious, 23, 122, 124–125
diuretics, 44
diverticulitis, 56
dopamine levels, 162
drugs
    driving and, 31

narcotics, 43
prescribed, 43–44
drug therapy, 1
dysgeria, 4, 17

Elder, Jocelyn, 176
environment, and life expectancy, 18, 21
enzymes, and free radicals, 10–11, 11
eugeria
    age at starting to prepare for, 3
    authors' success with program, 226–229
    beginning of period of, 16
    defined, xi, 16
    longevity and, 16–17
    prolonging, 17–18
Evans, Gary W., 83
exercise, 220–221. *See also* physical activity
    aerobic, 167–168
eye exams, 29
eye-lifts, 213, 214, 217, 218, 227, 229

face, 207–218
face-lifts, 213–218, 227, 229
facial aging, 207–218
    antidotes to, 209–212
    bone structure and, 212
    plastic surgery and, 212, 213–218
family relationships, 172
fasting, 13
fats, 59, 60, 139
    composition of, 61
    recommended intake, 62, 136
    saturated, 141–142
    watching intake of, 137
fatty acids, essential, 60–61
    adrenaline and, 63
    monounsaturated, 62, 63, 67, 139
    polyunsaturated, 20, 60–61, 62, 63, 67, 96–97
    saturated, 61, 63, 67, 139

supplements, 161
fiber, dietary, 55–56, 140
fifty-year-olds, 3
fish, 140, 146, 161, 165
    marinated, Tahitian style (recipe), 147
fish oils, 61, 161, 196
flavonoids, 143, 144, 155, 158, 195
fluoride, 87
folic acid. *See* vitamin B$_9$
Food and Drug Administration (FDA), 2, 90, 91
Food and Nutrition Board, 90, 149
foods. *See also* diet; nutrition
    animal products, 67
    to avoid (food don'ts), 141–142
    cholesterol in, 68
    cooking, 139, 142, 146
    eating slowly, 142, 148
    fried, 142
    natural, 192–193
    nutritive value of (table), 231–240
    organic, 141
    processed, 141
    recommended (food do's), 137–141, 145–146
    as risk factor, 47
Fossel, Michael, 121
Framingham study, 39–40, 65, 119, 226
free radicals
    and aging, 10–12, 152
    body's defense against, 153
    defined, 10
    LDL and, 66
    omega-6 oils and, 61, 67
    oxygen-based, 10–11
    pollution and, 45
    wrinkles and, 36
friends, 173
From Dream to Reality with Cosmetic Surgery (Lintilhac), 214
fruits, 137–138, 145

garlic, 138, 148
genetic clocks, 9, 121
genetic codes, 10
genetic inheritance, 3, 12, 69,
    120–123
genetic therapy, 123
Gerovital, 6, 166
ginkgo biloba, 164–165, 196
ginseng, 164, 196
glutathione, 156, 158
glutathione peroxydase, 11, 154, 156
glycation, 83
goals, importance of, 129
Goldstein, Joseph L., 66
growth hormone, 188–189
gynecological exams, 28

Hayflick, Leonard, 121
heart attack, 49, 55, 64, 65, 69, 119,
    131
  aspirin and, 184–185
  hormone replacement therapy
    and, 182
  wine and, 142–143
heart disease. See cardiovascular
    disease; heart attack
Henderson, B. E., 181–182
heredity. See genetic inheritance
high-density lipoproteins (HDL),
    65, 83, 142
HMG CoA reductase, 66–67
hobbies, 129
homocysteine, 65–66, 108, 111–112,
    163
hormone replacement therapy, 12,
    183, 184, 196, 222, 228
hormone treatments for eugeria,
    179–192
hyperglycemia, 53
hypertension, 30, 44, 141
  lifestyle adjustments and, 120
  obesity and, 49
  systolic, 119–120
hypoglycemia, 53

immune system
  aging and, 124–125
  strengthening, 125–127
  weakened, 124–127
impotence, treatment options,
    174–175, 187–188
independence, value of, 17
inflammation
  aspirin and, 185, 186–187
  free radicals caused by, 152
influenza, 125, 127
inheritance. See genetic inheritance
insomnia, 130, 163, 191
insulin, 12, 63, 83, 84
  diabetes and, 53–55
interests, 128–129
iodine, 81
ions, negative, 178
iron, 79–80
isolation, 130

kidney problems, 58, 59, 145

learning new skills, 172
lecithin, 116, 117, 163–164, 196
life expectancy. See also longevity
  cholesterol levels and, 70
  excess weight and, 48–49
  genetic clock and, 121
  in good health, 16–17
  projected, 15–17
lifestyle
  hypertension and, 120
  risk factors for disease, 29–31
linolenic acid, 126
Lintilhac, Jean Paul, ix–x, 2–3
Lintilhac, Simone, ix–x, 4–6, 14, 22,
    31, 45, 71–72, 145–146, 148,
    159–160, 170–171, 222–224,
    228–229
lipoproteins, 65, 66, 83, 143
liposuction, 220, 221–222
longevity, 15–22
  average, 15–16

factors related to, 18, 21
quiz, 19–20
low-density lipoproteins (LDL), 65,
66, 83, 143
lung X rays, 28–29
lycopene, 92, 154

magnesium, 78–79, 151–152, 163,
195
makeup, 223–224
malnutrition, 51
mammograms, 25, 28
mammoplasty, 221
manganese, 86–87
marital status of men, and life
expectancy, 18
massage, facial, 212
meat, red, 141–142
medical care, regular, 25–31. *See also*
tests, medical
medicine, alternative, on nutrition, 1
medicine, conventional, 29
on nutrition, 1
melatonin, 12, 163, 190–192, 196
memory, 117, 161–166
men
cosmetic surgery, 218
life expectancy, 15
marital status, and life expectancy,
18
sex life, 173–175
sexual dysfunction, treatment
options, 174–175, 187–188
testosterone replacement therapy,
187–188
menopause, 180–182
mental activity, 171–173
mental aging. *See* brain aging;
memory
methionine, 155, 196
minerals, 73–88. *See also specific*
minerals
antioxidants and, 158
trace elements, 80–88

mineral supplements, 51, 125,
148–149
advice to manufacturers, 160
choosing, 158–159
recommended intake, 151–152
USP standard, 150
moderation recommended, 3
moisturizers, 210–211
molybdenum, 88

narcotics, 43
nicotine, 37, 38–39
Niehans, Paul, 6, 193–194
nutrients, 51–68
assimilation of, 51
nutrition, 1 *See also* diet; nutrients
basic guidelines, 135–137
denutrition state, 161
malnutrition, 51
nutritive value of foods (table),
136, 231–240
reduced calorie program and, 13
special needs, 136
nutritive value of (table), 231–240

obesity, 30, 47–50, 145
olive oil, 139
omega-3 oils, 61, 62, 67, 140, 161,
165
omega-6 oils, 61, 62, 126, 161
oncogenes, 122–123
organic foods, 141
osteoporosis, 42, 180–181
oxidative stress, 159
oxygen-based free radicals, 10
ozone, 44–45

parathyroid glands, 76
Paris study, 63
Pauling, Linus, 116
phosphorus, 77–78
physical activity, 69, 128, 129,
167–171. *See also* exercise
caloric expenditure and, 48

Physical activity (*continued*)
 life expectancy and, 18
pineal gland, 190–191
pituitary gland, 11
plastic surgeons, 214–215, 217–218
plastic surgery
 of body, 219, 221–222
 facial (cosmetic), 212, 213–218
pollution, 98
 atmospheric, 44–45
potassium, 74
proanthocyanidols, 143
procaine, 166
progeria, 16
prostaglandins, 126
prostate cancer, 187
prostate exams, 28
proteins, 56–59
 recommended intake, 59, 136
 sources of, 57–58
provitamins, 92
pulse, testing, 25
pycnogenol, 158

Raben, S. M., 188
radiation, 152
 ionizing, 45
Retin-A, 211, 223
retinol. *See* vitamin A
retirement, 128, 129, 227
 suggested daily schedule, 197–199
REVES, 16
rheumatism, 49
risk factors. *See also specific risk factors,*
 e.g. alcohol consumption;
 obesity
 for cardiovascular disease, 30
 genetic inheritance, 120–124
 hypertension, 119–120
 idleness, 128–129
 immunity, weakened, 124–127
 lifestyle, 29–31
 related to nutrition, 47–72
 related to toxic substances, 35–45

retirement, 128
 stress, 127–128, 129–132
Robine, J. L., 161
routine, daily, 197–199

salt, 141
Sears, Barry, 67
sedentary lifestyle, 30, 128–129
selenium, 85–86, 158, 195
Selye, Hans, 129
serotonin, 104–105
sex life, 173–177
 of men, 173–175
 of women, 176
sixty-year-olds, 3
skin, 203–206
 aging of, 204–206
 of body, 219–224
 daily treatment, 223–224
 examining, 27
 facial, 207–211
 nightly treatment, 223
 polyunsaturated oils and, 60
 sagging, surgery for, 222
 smoking and, 36, 208
skin lesions, age-related, 205–206,
 211
 treatments for, 211
sleep disorders, 163
SMAS, 213
smoking. *See* also nicotine;
 tobacco
 quitting, 38–39
 wrinkles and, 36, 208
snacks, 137
sodium, 73–74
solitude, 172
soy, 138–139
 lecithin from, 117, 163–164
spas, 177–178
statines, 67
stress, 30
 causative factors, 130–131
 cholesterol levels and, 69

stress. (*continued*)
    oxidative, 159
    physical effects, 130
stress coping with, 131–132
stretching, 169–170
stroke, 23, 24, 55, 120, 182
    aspirin and, 184–185
    hormone replacement therapy
        182
    sulfur, 79
sun exposure, 208, 209–210, 219
sunscreens, 209–210
superoxide dismutase (SOD), 11, 81,
        87, 153
surgery, and obesity, 49
surgery, plastic. See cosmetic
surgery; plastic surgery

tai chi, 169, 227
tannins, 143, 144
T-cells, 124
tea, 137, 144
teeth, false, 212
telomeres, 9, 121
testosterone replacement therapy,
        187–188
tests, medical, 25–29
    annual, 27–29
thalassotherapy, 6, 177–178
thymus gland, 82, 124, 191
    as cell therapy, 125
thyroid gland, 81
thyroxin, 11–12
tobacco, 30, 35–39, 125, 130
tocopherols, 155. *See also* vitamin E
toxic substances, 21, 30, 35–45
    limiting exposure to, 35
trace elements, 80–88
triglycerides, 63
tryptophan, 104–105

ulcerative colitis, and nicotine, 37
United States Pharmacopoeia
    (USP), 91

uremia, 58
uric acid, 59, 71

vaccinations, 127
vegetables, 137–138, 145
vitamin(s), 88–117. *See also antioxi-*
    dants and *specific vitamins*
    deficiencies, 89–90 (*see also under*
        specific vitamins)
    fat-soluble, 91–100
    water-soluble, 91, 92, 100–116
vitamin A (retinol), 91–94, 151, 154
    Retin-A, 211, 223
vitamin B$_1$ (thiamin), 88, 100–102,
        152
vitamin B$_2$ (riboflavin), 102–103
vitamin B$_3$ (niacin), 103–105
vitamin B$_4$ (pantothenic acid),
        105–107
vitamin B$_6$ (pyridoxine), 66, 107–109,
        152
vitamin B$_7$. See choline
vitamin B$_8$ (biotin), 109–110,
        125, 152, 163
vitamin B$_9$ (folic acid), 66, 108,
        110–112, 152, 163
vitamin B$_{12}$ (cyanocobalamine), 66,
        112–114, 152, 163
vitamin C (ascorbic acid), 97,
        114–116, 155, 159, 195
vitamin D, 77, 94–96, 151, 158, 210
vitamin E, 85, 86, 96–98, 139, 155,
        158, 159, 195, 196
vitamin F, 60
vitamin K, 99–100
vitamin supplements, 51, 125,
        148–149
    advice to manufacturers, 160
    choosing, 158–159
    recommended intake, 149–150,
        151, 152, 158
    USP standard, 150

Walford, Roy, 13, 14, 67, 225

walking, 167, 168
water, 52
weight, 26
    caloric intake and, 51
    excess, 47–50
    fluctuations in, 50
    ideal, 135–136
    loss of, 50
    maintaining, 135–136
weight training, 168–169
wines, 142–144, 148
women
    cosmetic surgery, 218
    hormone replacement therapy,
        180–182
    life expectancy, 15

life expectancy, factors related to,
    18, 21
sex life, 176
work, and life expectancy, 18. *See also*
    retirement
wrinkles
    dieting and, 209
    facial exercises and, 208–209
    free radicals and, 36
    sun and, 208
    treatments for, 211

Yen, Samuel, 190
yoga, 169

zinc, 81–82, 86, 126, 151